MORE *from* LIFE

Malcolm Bronte-Stewart

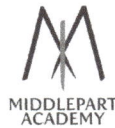

MIDDLEPART
ACADEMY

Published in 2023 by Middlepart Academy Ltd.

ISBN Paperback: 978-1-7394485-0-9
Ebook: 978-1-7394485-1-6

A CIP catalogue copy of this book can be found in the British Library.

Published with the help of Indie Authors World
www.indieauthorsworld.com

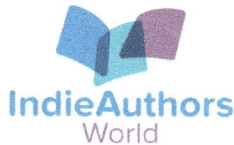

IndieAuthors
World

To Daune, Kate, Jamie, Rob, Kylie, Rudy, Aurelia and Felix.

Acknowledgements

I would like to acknowledge the significant contribution made by John Welsh to the early development and testing of the More Life approach and thank my wife, sisters and children for the support they have given. I would also like to acknowledge Kev Brown for the inspiration he provides.

Contents

Conclusions

Why did I write this book?

I felt reasonably healthy and well until I was 52. I didn't really think about it. I had always had an active life, cross country running, playing rugby and hockey, winning swimming galas, teaching canoeing and skiing, running an outward-bound course, trout fishing, working as an oilfield geologist, then systems analyst, before settling down. My wife and I divided our time mostly between work as university lecturers and running our farm and equitation centre. My kids were independent and doing well.

Then a horse-riding accident fractured my pelvis. It had to be repaired, surgically, with metal plates and screws. Suddenly I was housebound, no more horse riding, skiing, visits to the gym, I couldn't even take the dogs for a walk for a while. I worked from home, drinking red wine became a habit and I started to eat too much cheesy, salty, packaged, processed, convenience foods and tasty BBQ sausages, bacon rolls, white bread and ham sandwiches, croissants, pepperoni pizza and ready meals. Within a year I had gained well over a stone (8 kgs) in weight, become anxious, stressed about work, and was unable to sleep through the night. I started to worry about my health. From time to time I had frightening bouts of palpitations and was shocked to learn that I had developed high cholesterol levels and was classified as pre-diabetic. These seemed important warnings and I began to read extensively to learn about health and wellbeing.

My father died when I was 11. I was aware that his nutrition and heart disease research had been cutting edge and I was suddenly embarrassed to realise I knew very little about his work. I searched for, and read for the first time, medical science papers he published in the 1950s. He pioneered research in the role of cholesterol in the causation of atheroma and the connection between salt intake and hypertension. He had examined and compared the Standard American Diet (full of animal fat) with the traditional diets of Japan (vegetables and fish, little meat) and South Africa (almost entirely plant-based) and highlighted the apparent stark differences in atherosclerosis and cardio vascular health. He investigated the heart health of bus drivers and bus conductors to try to learn what effect, if any, physical activity and stress made to heart disease rates. Research that Nathan Pritikin, Dean Ornish and Caldwell Esselstyn continued, showing that Cardio Vascular Disease and other chronic illnesses can be prevented, halted and sometimes reversed by changes in diet and lifestyle. My mother worked as an eye doctor in the NHS until she was 70. Her research into scurvy and the complications of diabetic eye disease confirmed the importance of nutrition. The evidence had been staring me in the face for years. I started to understand why our family meals had been so plant-based.

Working in a university made it easier to access up-to-date, scientific research on staying healthy and sift good evidence from bad (I am sad to say that there is a lot of nonsense and vested interest misinformation out there). My family doctor wrote a prescription for statins but offered little advice.

I started to ask questions and found that many of my friends, colleagues and clients suffered from an astonishing wealth of symptoms and health worries. 2 had experienced "minor" strokes, 1 had had a heart attack, 3 were already classified as having type two diabetes, 2 had cancer, many of them were taking medication to lower their blood pressure or thin their blood viscosity, 2 were off work with stress, one was taking 28 pills every day, and several had given up exercising for one reason or another. Most of them told me that they had little warning or knowledge of these problems before they occurred. I was surprised that, generally speaking, they seemed to know very little about their own health and had been given few, if any, ways to track their own condition, other than to agree to regular blood tests and to attend occasional hospital assessments. It was as if they had accepted that this was their destiny – their inevitable fate, so be it, what could they do, this was genetic and or written in the stars.

I wanted to help. I was convinced that many people could live a healthier life. I was keen to believe that, given a chance, our bodies will heal themselves. After all, my father and others had been pointing this out for decades. But how many people know how to achieve a *More* (healthy and happy) *Life?* And how do they assess their own evolving health status or spot trends?

Frustrated by the apparent lack of useful, quantifiable, health and wellbeing tests I began to collect and create assessments that could be used to measure a wide variety of evaluations. Professional experts such as doctors, psychologists, psychiatrists, dietitians, nutritionists, physiotherapists, personal trainers, dentists, optometrists, chiropractors, osteopaths, podiatrists, acupuncturists, meditation tutors and alternative medicine advocates focus on divergent knowledge bases and disciplines which are often quite distinct and poorly connected. My understanding of Systems Theory helped me to search for a broad view and prompted questions. I began to think of health and well-being as a complex interaction of many parts and connected (physical and mental, objective and subjective) components and wondered to what extent these could be quantified and assessed in ways that were meaningful and reasonably easy to obtain. It seemed useful to try to group and capture these issues under 4 main headings (systems within a bigger system), Mind, Body, Exercise and Nutrition. I developed a set of tests to help measure aspects and views of each of these parts.

Teaming up with John Welsh, the owner of a strength and conditioning gym, we set up a 7-day challenge named "Life Number" which invited people to take a range of assessments, each of which was scored / quantified numerically, to generate a total score out of 240, which represented their Life Number. 17 individuals returned a week after their first assessments, having followed a program of suggestions and rules (to keep to a plant-based diet, avoid alcohol and tobacco, do some exercise every day and make efforts to connect with and look after other people). All the participants achieved better results in the second set of tests than the first, on average they increased their Life Number scores by 10% in just one week.

This 7-day challenge shows how quickly we can improve our overall health and well-being. (The experiment was written up, presented at a conference and published in a peer-reviewed academic journal named the Systemist, volume 43(2), December 2022). The COVID-19 pandemic closed all gyms preventing us from taking the initiative any further in the in-person form. However, I was impressed that the Life Number idea seemed to work well so I set myself the challenge to produce it as a more complete set of self-assessed indicators – thus the idea for a book.

It is almost 20 years since my horse-riding accident. The changes I made to my lifestyle since then have made a big difference. The palpations and feelings of anxiety are gone, BMI and body fat are under control, cholesterol and blood glucose levels are normal, I'm back to riding horses, doing farm work, taking the dogs for forest and beach walks, and going on long cycle rides. I sleep well, eat well and feel good. I track my numbers. I get More out of Life and hopefully give *More From Life*.

Chapter 1

Introduction

How do you feel?

How fit, healthy and happy are you at the moment?

When was the last time you had a comprehensive check-up or took stock of your overall well-being?

Do you know how you rate in the important indicators of health?

How, and how quickly, can you improve your health?

What aspects of your life should you pay most attention to?

Would you like to find answers to these questions?

What is this book about?

Based on the latest research, this book aims to help you to investigate and enhance your health and well-being. It provides you with ways to measure your status. It offers challenges and guidelines. It includes the most extensive and comprehensive set of health, well-being and transformation assessments ever.

These days there is so much advice, pseudoscience and conflicting information out there, telling us what to do and how to live our lives. How does anyone make sense of it all? Lifestyle promotions and healthy living adverts bombard us with suggestions, claims and questionable data. Government campaigns often target only one or two factors at a time without giving us enough understanding of how to fit recommendations together. Most family doctors have been trained to deal with ill health once it occurs or develops, rather than anticipate and prevent it.

The myth persists that effective treatments for many health problems are bound to involve drugs, technology, surgery, or even something expensive, under trial and hard to get. Some people find it difficult to believe that the choices we make every day, (such as what we eat, how much we exercise and keep active, how we deal with stress, the quality of our relationships, the impacts of environmental pollutants, and whether we smoke or drink too much alcohol), make a remarkably powerful difference to our health and well-being. Most of the killer diseases are caused by these choices. We can increase our healthy longevity by over a decade.

We can distinguish two types of *longevity:* life-span = how long we live (*More Life*), and health-span = our quality of life (*More From Life*). The term *biological age* is often used to refer to estimates of the health and vitality of one or more of a person's 78 organs (eg their heart, liver, kidneys, arteries, lungs and skin). Unlike *chronological age*, which is determined solely by the number of years someone has been alive. Biological age takes into account the wear and tear that the body has experienced over time, as well as any genetic factors that may affect health.

Adopting a healthy diet that is rich in fruits, vegetables, and other nutrient-dense foods can help reduce inflammation and improve overall health. Regular exercise has numerous benefits for physical and mental well-being, including reducing the risk of chronic diseases and improving cognitive function. Other lifestyle factors that can help to slow down the aging process include getting enough sleep, drinking plenty of water, nurturing thriving relationships and avoiding harmful behaviours.

Micro-Morts and Micro-Lives

The Micro-Mort (MM) concept was invented as a way to measure or quantify the risk of activities and behaviours. A Micro-Mort is supposed to be equivalent to a one in a million chance of dying. So, for example riding a motorcycle 100 miles = 18 MMs, cycling the same distance = 5 MMs, smoking 14 cigarettes = 10 MMs, a general anaesthetic and skydiving both = 10MMs.

A Micro-Life (ML) on the other hand is a unit of risk that represents a half an hour change of life expectancy. It is supposed to be an approximate but reasonable comparison between the relative amounts of certain risks, converting them into more tangible time units. One Micro-Life is the loss or gain of 30 minutes of life, because 1,000,000 half hours (57 years) corresponds roughly to an adult lifetime. For example:

- eating 5 servings of fruit and vegetables gives you +4 ML (ie 4 x 30 minutes = plus 2 hours of life),

- smoking 15 to 24 cigarettes gives -10 ML (ie -10 x 30 minutes = minus 5 hours),

- the first drink (of 10 g alcohol) = +1 ML, each subsequent drink (up to 6) = −½ ML,

- for every 5 units above a BMI of 22.5 each day = -3 ML,

- for every 2 hours sedentary, watching a screen = −1 ML,

- the first 20 minutes of moderate exercise = +2 ML, the subsequent 40 minutes of moderate exercise = +1 ML;

- every portion of red meat, (85 g, 3 oz) = -1 ML,

- every 2 to 3 cups of coffee = +1 ML.

So, unhealthy ways cost Micro-Lives. A 20-a-day habit may accelerate you towards your death at 29 hours for each day you live. The big difference between Micro-Morts and Micro-Lives is that if you survive the motorbike trip your Micro-Morts are forgotten and you start the next day with a clean slate, but if you smoke, drink lots of alcohol, do no exercise and live on a fast-food diet, your Micro-Lives accumulate and build every day. The good news is, however, that the converse is also true, adopting a healthier way of life adds Micro-Lives.

The Interheart study, which followed 30,000 men and women in 52 countries, found that certain, well-known factors accounted for 95% of the risk of heart attack. These are: poor diet, smoking, diabetes, obesity, high blood pressure, little physical activity, high cholesterol levels, excessive alcohol consumption, and psychosocial issues such as stress and depression.

The World Health Organisation defines health as "a state of complete physical, mental and social well-being, and not merely the absence of disease". How healthy you are and how you feel depend on many different issues, and we know that these different issues interact and affect each other. For example, doing more exercise may help you to lose some excess weight, feel happier and more confident and give you more strength and vitality.

Eating a better diet can prevent the early onset of (and sometimes reverse) chronic conditions such as high blood pressure, heart disease, diabetes, certain cancers and many other diseases. Actively looking after your mental health can make you more relaxed, positive, in control, enthusiastic and good to know. Paying attention to most or all of these areas (your exercise, health, mind and diet) tends to have beneficial effects in multiple ways, which can build on, and boost, each other.

The More From Life approach

You can dip randomly into this book, try a few tests or have a look at some of the topics, or follow the chapters sequentially – they are organised in a structure to take you through a progression of stages. After the introduction we look at recent research evidence on aspects of health and well-being – how unhealthy are we and why we need to learn more about measuring and monitoring our own health. Next the book provides five different sets of assessments, followed by a 7-day challenge. The last sections of the book take a longer-term view of ways and means to improve and maintain health and well-being.

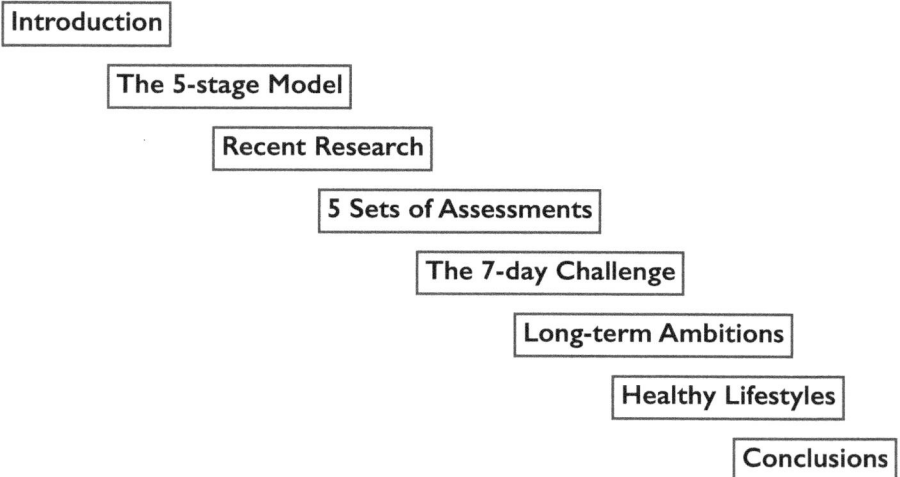

Introduction

    The 5-stage Model

        Recent Research

            5 Sets of Assessments

                The 7-day Challenge

                    Long-term Ambitions

                        Healthy Lifestyles

                            Conclusions

The *More From Life* assessments are designed to help you to figure out your present overall wellness from several different perspectives, and let you build a more complete picture of your health and well-being, so that you can see which aspects you may want to work on. The idea is to look at 5 important areas using insightful and established tests, measurements and assessments so that you can learn about yourself, discover your scores and figure out what to do.

So what are the **5 areas** we are going to investigate and evaluate?

1) The Mind

In this quadrant the aim is to explore personal mental wellbeing with a set of questionnaires. Research shows that we need to take care of our mental health every bit as much as our physical health. We should give ourselves time to relax and have fun, we should try to boost our happiness, engage with our friends and family, look after our work–life balance and have purpose in our lives. The questions are designed to help you to assess, and give scores to, the way you feel at the moment, your present state of mind. How's life? How happy are you? Do you feel good? Are you satisfied with the way things are? The sets of questions are based on tried and tested tools and resources that are often used by scientists and psychologists.

There are four sets of questionnaires (that contain 10 questions each) which invite you to respond, using Likert scales, which number, between 0 and 10, you think is the most appropriate answer for each question. You can return to the questions and your answers in a few days to see if you still feel the same.

The 4 questionnaires ask about: How relaxed or stressed you have been; Your happiness and self esteem; Your work / life balance and Your relationships and personal life.

2) The Body

The body quadrant aims to focus on measurements that assess aspects of a person's medical health. Individuals can carry out these tests themselves and or ask another person to help. The assessments fall into groups:

- Starter background questions. 20 yes or no questions to explore some fundamental issues.

- Reaction Time and Thinking / Memory tests. Two interesting and fun assessments that aim to establish how fast you can react to a stimulus and how effective your thinking and memory are.

- Body Composition. Obesity is one of the root causes of many diseases and visceral fat can be dangerous. The World Health Organization (WHO) classifies obesity as one of the leading preventable causes of death worldwide. Obesity is associated with a reduction in quality of life, poorer mental health outcomes, obstructive sleep apnoea, increases in "bad" cholesterol, as well as cardiovascular disease, stroke, certain cancers and diabetes. Individuals record details such as height, waist circumference and weight and figure out their waist to height, BMI and visceral fat calculations.

- Cardio Vascular health. Blood pressure measurements, SpO^2 (oxygen levels) and resting pulse rates are regarded as useful indicators of illness. Devices can be purchased that allow individuals to do frequent tests of these parameters, note what times of the day and what circumstances cause them to fluctuate but also make it easier for people to see trends.

- Blood Tests. Another pair of tests that are commonly carried out during medical examinations are Cholesterol and Blood Glucose level assessments. Basic blood test kits that allow people to test themselves and monitor their status can be purchased in most high street chemist shops. While these tests may not be as accurate as those conducted by medical professionals, they can provide useful indications.

- Poo / faeces. Poo or faeces are the remains of the food that bacteria have fermented in the gut and that the intestine did not digest or absorb. Bacterial biomass makes up 25% to 50% of the dry weight of poop. The rest is mostly undigested carbohydrate, fibre, protein, fat, and dead epithelial cells from the walls of the gastrointestinal tract. We should monitor our poo production and check its colour, texture and frequency.

More From Life includes a wealth of tables to evaluate and score the results of these assessments so that individuals can give themselves points for each of the tests.

3) Exercise, Strength and Fitness

The benefits of regular exercise and physical activity are well known and include:

- boosts energy, strength, resilience and endurance;
- improves mood;
- promotes better sleep;
- combats certain health conditions and diseases;
- eliminates toxins when we sweat;
- helps to manage weight;
- strengthens bones and muscles;
- improves cognitive function;
- can be fun and social,
- improves physical appearance,
- boosts confidence and self-esteem; and
- can put the spark back into sex life.

The NHS puts it this way: *"Exercise is the miracle cure we've always had, but for too long we've neglected to take our recommended dose. Our health is now suffering as a consequence. Whatever your age, there's strong scientific evidence that being physically active can help you lead a healthier and happier life. People who exercise regularly have a lower risk of developing many long-term (chronic) conditions"*. For most healthy adults, the NHS recommends at least 150 minutes a week of moderate aerobic activity or 75 minutes a week of vigorous aerobic activity a week, plus strength training for all the major muscle groups at least twice a week.

The Exercise / Fitness quadrant is gauged by a range of assessments including:

- Functional Movement, evaluated using a 5 part test in which posture control, core stability and mobility are assessed with: Overhead Bodyweight Squat, Shoulder and Thoracic Mobility and Straight Leg Raise.

- Daily activity is assessed with an average-number-of-steps-per-day count.
- Flexibility and balance are assessed by a sit and reach test and a one-leg balance test.
- Aerobic fitness is assessed with a 5km walk or run and the VO2 Max type of Step test.
- Strength and power are measured using several well-known tests: press ups, plank, standing long jump and quadriceps wall squat.

4) Nutrition and Diet

Health authorities such as the NHS, the Eatwell Guide and the USDA as well as extensively researched studies such as the Lancet EAT Commission and NutritionFacts.org recommend that we should stop consuming refined, processed foods and adopt a predominately whole-food, plant-based diet. Man-made and processed foods produce different effects to whole foods / foods in their original form. The bulk of our diet should consist of organic: leafy green and colourful vegetables, fruits, legumes, seeds, starchy vegetables, nuts and whole grains, that provide sufficient fibre, vitamins, minerals, antioxidants, alkaline-forming foods, electrolytes, essential fats, iron, calcium, protein, carbohydrates, raw food and phytonutrients.

Dr. Michael Greger recommend that we consume: "a minimum of three servings of beans (legumes), one serving of berries, three servings of other fruits, one serving of cruciferous vegetables, two servings of greens, two servings of other veggies, one serving of flaxseeds, one serving of nuts and seeds, one serving of herbs and spices, three servings of whole grains, and five servings of beverages" each day.

An easy way to think about what you should and should not consume is to use a traffic light analogy.

1. Green Light = Items we should eat, good food.

2. Amber Light = Items we should limit our consumption of, moderate and be cautious about.

3. Red Light = Items we should avoid, substances that, over time, are likely to be poisonous and bad for us.

5) Central Issues (the Fifth Quadrant).

While the first four *More From Life* sections, mentioned so far, have many different parts and assessments the fifth (central) one has far fewer. Time and again research shows that smoking, alcohol consumption, inadequate hydration and lack of sleep are associated with poor Healthy Life Expectancy. People who do not smoke, moderate their alcohol intake, drink enough water and get plenty of sleep every day tend to feel better and live longer.

- Smoking is probably the most significant single lifestyle factor of all, it causes almost countless chronic diseases and health problems, quitting can generate rapid benefits.

- Alcohol is another modifiable habit and excessive boozing (more than a unit a day) can potentially cause physical, mental and social damage.

- It has become clear that drinking enough water is crucial to sustain a healthy body, yet it seems that few people know if they are dehydrated.

- Research confirms that restful sleep is essential at all ages. Sleep restores the mind and the body, and is good for almost every mental and physiological system we rely on. Guidelines advise that most healthy adults need between 7 and 9 hours of restful sleep per night.

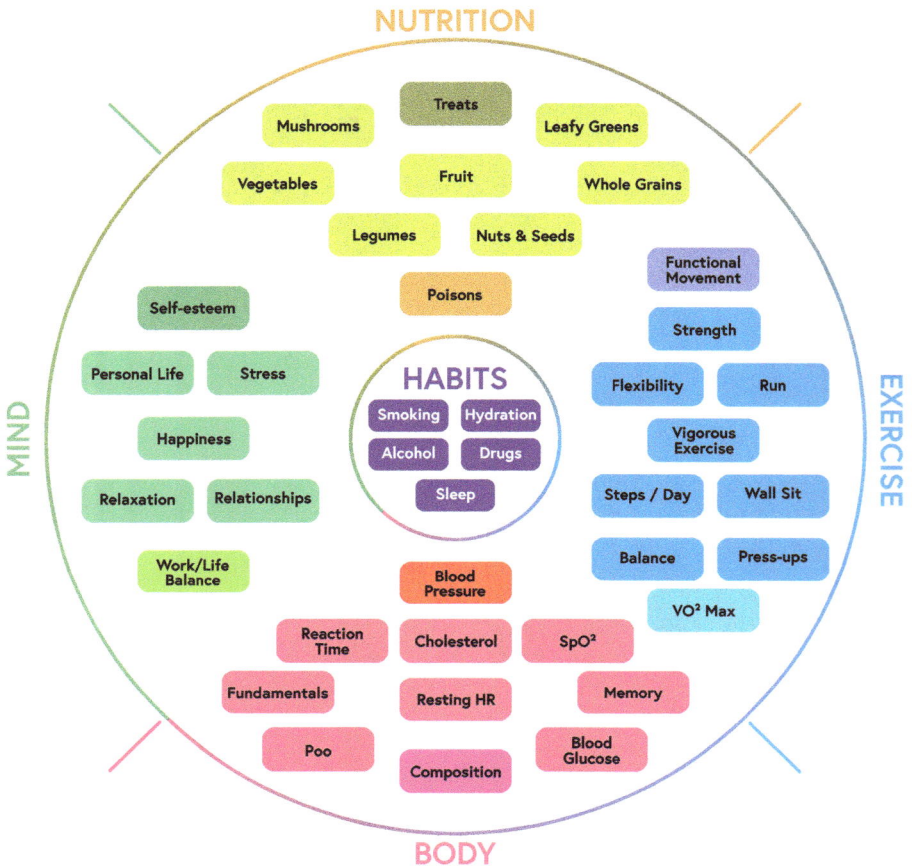

The circular *More From Life* model displays representations of the evaluations and assessments in the four quarters that represent the main elements of the More From Life approach: Mind, Body, Exercise, and Nutrition and a Central part that contains other important considerations.

These 5 health and well-being sections contain scored questions, tests and measurements that each amount to 100 points and contribute to the maximum number or total that an individual can achieve, a score out of 500. You can do the tests and assessments and see how you get on – how many points out of 500 will you get?

The *More From Life* approach has been designed as a set of well-being evaluations and indicators that help to provide a good general overview.

You can try them in any order, take your time and do as many as you feel like, building an overall picture.

You don't have to feel great to make a start but you have to make a start to feel great.

One Week to a Better You

Your *More From Life* scores will change over time – as you make changes to your lifestyle – you can track your progress and see how you are doing in a holistic way. Research shows that we can improve our scores (the indicators of our health) remarkably and surprisingly quickly. To help you achieve this, chapter 8 provides eight rules and guidelines to follow to complete the *One Week Challenge*. These include avoiding alcohol and smoking, eating a wholefood plant-based diet, being active and doing 10,000 steps a day, trying to do 10 minutes of meditation, mindfulness or yoga a day, and making efforts to be a good example, nurture relationships and enjoy your world. After 7-days you test yourself again and see what your new scores are and where the differences are. What have you learned? Do you feel healthier and happier?

Once you have completed the *One Week Challenge* you can go on to set longer-term ambitions, decide what you want to achieve next, live a healthier life and try the *7 Week* and then the *7 month challenges*.

Please note that the suggestions, comments, opinions and tests in this book should not be regarded or taken as medical advice. The assessments have been designed for reasonably healthy adults. While it is unlikely that any of the ideas and proposals presented will cause harm, to be safe, you should consult your doctor before beginning some of the *More From Life* assessments, especially if you have any significant health issues or conditions. The book is for informational and educational purposes only and the authors do not accept any responsibilities for any real or perceived liabilities or damages resulting from the information and evaluations it contains.

Readiness Questionnaire

The *More From Life* assessments are very safe for most people. Some people, however, should check with health professionals before they take part. These questions have been designed to identify the small number of adults for whom the tests and evaluations may be inappropriate or those who should have medical advice concerning the type of activity most suitable for them.

Answer the following questions:

1. Has a medically qualified doctor ever said that you have a heart condition and that you should only do physical activity recommended by a doctor?

2. Do you have, or have you recently felt, pain in your chest when you do physical activity?

3. Do you lose your balance because of dizziness or do you ever lose consciousness?

4. Do you have a bone or joint problem that could be made worse by a change in your physical activity?

5. Is your doctor currently prescribing drugs for your blood pressure or heart condition?

6. Do you know of any other reason why you should not do physical activity?

If you answered YES to one or more of these questions, are older than 40 years of age and have been inactive or are concerned about your health, consult a physician before taking a fitness test or substantially increasing your physical activity. You should ask for a medical clearance along with information about specific exercise limitations you may have. In most cases, you will still be able to do any type of activity you want as long as you adhere to some guidelines.

If you answered NO to all the questions, you can be reasonably confident that you can perform the assessments in this book safely and have a low risk of having any medical complications from exercise. It is probably a good idea to start slowly and increase gradually. It may also be helpful to have a fitness assessment with a personal trainer in order to determine what to do and where to begin.

If you are not feeling well because of a temporary illness, such as flu or a fever, wait until you feel better to begin exercising. If you are, or may be, pregnant, talk with your doctor before you become more active.

If your health changes, in a way that you would answer "YES" to any of the above questions, talk to a doctor or health professional, and ask whether you should change any of the plan.

Recommended Equipment

Many of the evaluations and tests in this book do not require special or expensive equipment. To complete all the assessments, you will need the following items:

- Notebook and or diary
- Pens or pencils
- Smart Watch* and or stopwatch
- Modern weighing machine*
- Cholesterol tester*
- Blood pressure monitor*
- Pulse oximeter / Fingertip SpO2 meter*
- Tape measure
- Ruler (wooden or plastic measuring device about 30cms long)
- Broom handle or stick
- Masking tape
- Pack of playing cards

(* = discussed in chapter 11).

You

Want to give it a try? Start your journey to a better understanding of an approach to improving your health and well-being, using the *More From Life* method, that is personalised and made to measure for you.

Name:

Address and / or postcode:

Month and Year of birth:

Height:

Gender:

Notes on why you want to try the One Week Challenge:

Important Medical History / Injuries / Test results:

Chapter 2

Background

Healthy Living Expectancy and Chronic Disease

Healthy Living Expectancy (HLE) is an estimate of how many years an individual can expect to live in 'very good' or 'good' general health, based on how individuals perceive their state of health at the time of completing an annual population survey. Figures show that in some parts of the developed world the HLE is only 55 years.

Many chronic diseases are increasing. World Health Organisation figures suggest that 108 million people suffered from Diabetes in 1980, but by 2014 it had become 422 million. Diabetes.co.uk estimates that 4.9 million people in the UK have type 2 with almost 1 million more undiagnosed and 13.6 million at increased risk. They estimate that this disease already accounts for around 10% of the NHS budget. 42% of adults in the USA are obese and 86% of them have at least one illness. 7.6 million people are living with Cardio Vascular Disease (CVD) in the UK. Someone dies of CVD every 3 minutes and strokes occur every 5 minutes. There are over 375,000 new cancer cases and around 167,000 cancer deaths in the UK every year, it is estimated that about 40% of these may be preventable. 68% of men and 60% of women in the UK are overweight or obese.

It appears that many people are living with debilitating illness and chronic conditions from quite an early age and research shows that this need not be the case. Lifestyle Medicine is evidence-based, clinical care that supports behaviour change through person-centred techniques to improve mental wellbeing, social connection, healthy eating, physical activity, sleep and minimisation of harmful substances and behaviours.

Prime causes of ill health

The Global Burden of Diseases, Injuries, and Risk Factors Study estimated the burden of mortality and disability attributable to dietary risks across 195 countries and territories was huge: 11 million deaths and 255 million years lost in disability and premature death.

U.S. health care spending grew 9.7% in 2020 reaching $4.1 trillion or $12,530 per person. As a share of the nation's Gross Domestic Product, health spending accounted for 19.7%. Despite this, each year around a million Americans experience their first heart attack or stroke; a million get diabetes; a million get cancer and during the last 100 years, US adult obesity appears to have increased from about 1 in 30 to 1 in 3 people. Over 20 years ago it was estimated that Americans were spending $33 billion per year on weight loss products, yet from 1999 to 2017 U.S. obesity prevalence increased and among 49 OECD countries the U.S. ranks 31st for life expectancy at birth.

These rather astonishing figures and trends may be explained partly by the findings of the American Institute for Cancer Research's ninth Cancer Risk Awareness Survey which found that fewer than half of Americans recognise that: diets low in vegetables, fruits and fibre; the consumption of red meat; drinking alcohol and insufficient physical activity all have a clear link to cancer development. Furthermore, awareness of other established cancer risk factors, like obesity and processed meat, is alarmingly low.

It is likely that much of the suffering and healthcare costs caused by chronic conditions can be reduced. Michael Greger claims that almost all of the top 15 killer diseases can be treated, prevented and sometimes reversed by changes in lifestyle.

In fact, "lifestyle" is known to be the leading cause of death. There is overwhelming evidence that a few behavioural factors significantly impact our health, wellbeing and enjoyment of a long active life. As long ago as 2002, Walter Willett, (Professor of Epidemiology and Nutrition at Harvard) noted that genes do not drive most chronic diseases. On the contrary, the risk of developing diabetes, heart disease, cancer, and autoimmunity is largely due to other factors. He went on to state that at least 70% of cases of stroke and colon cancer, over 80% of coronary heart disease and over 90% of type 2 diabetes cases are avoidable. He suggested that there should be more focus on the factors that are under the individual's control.

A study published in 2022 in the Lancet shows that physical inactivity is an important modifiable risk factor for non-communicable diseases and mental health conditions. The authors used the most recent health and economic data evidence available for disease outcomes in 194 countries including cases of coronary heart disease, stroke, type 2 diabetes, hypertension, cancer (breast, colon, bladder, endometrial, oesophageal, gastric, and renal), dementia, and depression in adults. The authors calculate that 499·2 million new cases of preventable major illness and chronic disease will occur globally by 2030 if the prevalence of physical inactivity does not change. The paper suggests that the global cost of physical inactivity will be $47·6 billion per year.

A 2021 report from the Cleveland Clinic states that 90% of the 18 million heart disease cases worldwide could be prevented by people adopting a healthier diet, doing regular exercise, and not smoking. The American College of Lifestyle Medicine notes 6 important considerations: nutrition, exercise, stress management, sleep, healthy relationships and toxins such as tobacco and alcohol. Research by the U.S. Burden of Disease Collaborators confirms that the leading risk factors related to disability-adjusted life-years were dietary risks, tobacco smoking, high body mass index, high blood pressure, high fasting plasma glucose, physical inactivity, and alcohol use.

A study of 23,153 German participants, aged 35 to 65, showed that those who had never smoked, had a BMI less than 30, a high intake of fruits, vegetables and whole-grains, low meat consumption, and did 3 ½ or more hours a week of physical activity had a 78% lower risk of developing a chronic disease (diabetes = 93%; myocardial infarction = 81%; stroke = 50%; and cancer = 36%).

Research that followed around 170,000 men and women for over 30 years found that those who had a healthy diet, did not smoke, drank alcohol in moderation, had a low BMI and were physically active, cut their risk of getting cancer by 65% and their risk of developing CVD by 82%. What is more, people who switch, mid-life, to a moderately healthy lifestyle (regular exercise, not smoking, a BMI of 18.5 to 29.9, and five or more fruits and vegetables eaten daily), "experience a prompt benefit of lower rates of cardiovascular disease and mortality."

To ensure a diverse gut microbiome, which helps to reduce inflammation and improve overall health, we should aim to eat around 30 different sources of real food each week. Real food means something that grows, not a packet or meal of something with 30 different chemicals in it. Consuming a wide variety of different fruit, vegetables, beans, nuts, seeds, and fermented foods each week has proven benefits for improving gut health.

Lessons from the Blue Zones

Aging / senescence is a normal part of life but we can slow it down and prevent the premature development of many age-related diseases by adopting a healthy lifestyle.

Dan Buettner and the Blue Zone study team investigated 5 places in the world in which people not only live far longer than average, but also remain active and productive into their 90s and beyond. Buettner looked for common characteristics and reported that, despite the distances between these places, the communities seem to have many lifestyle factors in common. He pointed to the apparent importance of:

- adopting a 95% to 100% plant-based diet (food should be whole, fresh, nutritious, unprocessed and include: beans, fruit, veg, nuts and berries. The consumption of meat, dairy, eggs, sugar and fish should be avoided or reduced),

- drinking lots of water,

- reducing stress,

- sleeping well,

- nurturing your social circle and improving relationships, (connecting and belonging, keeping in touch with family and friends),

- having purpose and responsibilities (keeping busy, useful and or important),
- being kind / nice, (giving, doing favours),
- moderating alcohol intake,
- not being overweight and
- staying active most of the day.

Lifestyle Medicine

The Ornish Reversal Program (UnDo It) is the first approach that is proven scientifically to reverse heart disease. Ornish suggests / demands that individuals adopt a healthy lifestyle by optimising four key areas:

a) What you eat - low-fat, whole foods, plant-based diet;

b) How much you move - at least 30 minutes of exercise each day;

c) How you manage stress - practice stress management techniques; and

d) How much love and support you have - active engagement in supportive relationships.

Backed by years of peer-reviewed evidence, Ornish has shown that adopting these guidelines reduces heart disease and can reverse type 2 diabetes, high cholesterol, obesity, high blood pressure and depression in as few as nine weeks, as well as prevent cancers and slow the aging process. The Ornish Lifestyle Program costs about $10,000, it consists of two 4 hour sessions per week for 9 weeks; for a total of 72 hours. Sessions include exercise, stress management, nutrition, and group support. Medicare and other medical insurance companies now cover this Lifestyle Medicine Program for reversing chronic disease because it achieves better clinical outcomes, larger cost savings, less surgical intervention and greater adherence than other options.

Those doctors and health professionals who practice *lifestyle medicine* can have a powerful influence on peoples' lives and help them to avoid premature illness. It has been said that many health care systems are at the limits of sustainability and in some cases on the verge of failure and or bankruptcy. So it is also important to consider the economic and organisational benefits of prevention-based lifestyle medicine. Many causes of pain, suffering, disability and death could be reduced if healthy lifestyle choices were promoted. Lifestyle medicine should be the primary approach to the management and prevention of chronic conditions.

Healthcare

Generally speaking, the UK's National Health Service (NHS) does not follow Lifestyle Medicine guidelines. It focusses on looking after people once they are ill rather than health promotion. It deals with health and well-being issues after they develop or occur. Non-emergency patients may only have a few minutes to explain their concerns, if they can get an appointment. GPs / family doctors often deal with symptoms, not underlying causes, temporary fixes may be prescribed, and serious illness may be caught late or go unrecognised. Doctors seldom have time to ask about nutrition, mental well-being and exercise. During their University course, they are given very little information about the importance of diet for general health; they are trained primarily to spot patterns and symptoms, recommend drugs and carry out surgical interventions, rather than investigate aspects of, give advice about, and source facilities for, holistic treatments and lifestyle medicine approaches.

The Royal College of General Practitioners, reporting the results of a survey of GPs in 2022, stated that 23% were so stressed that they could not cope on most or every day, 80% expect working in general practice to get worse over the next few years and 42% of GPs in England are likely to leave the profession within the next 5 years. 68% of GPs say they don't have enough time to adequately assess and treat patients during appointments and 65% say that patient safety is being compromised due to appointments being too short. Despite an agreement that 6,000 more GPs are needed, there are said to be 1,850 fewer fully qualified FTE GPs in 2022 than there were in 2015. Some estimates suggest that the UK is short of about 10,000 doctors and 50,000 nurses. The chair of the RCGP Council, Professor Martin Marshall, said that *"General practice is significantly understaffed, underfunded, and overworked and this is impacting on the care and services we're able to deliver to patients. The system is close to collapse".*

It is suggested that there have been 3 eras in medicine. Era 1 began in prehistoric times and could be characterised as an art, often having links to superstition, local culture, religious beliefs and philosophical ideas. For example, a witch doctor or physician may use magic, herbs, chanting or bloodletting in hope of a cure. Less than 200 years ago theories of science took over in era 2. Advances in understanding germs, bacteriology, vaccines, antibiotics and pharmaceutical drugs revolutionised medicine. Randomised control trials research produced rapid progress in the accuracy and effectiveness of diagnosis and treatment. We are moving towards the 3rd era in which personalised medicine will become more popular. Innovations including DNA sequencing, gene mapping and therapy, stem cell therapy, and wireless health monitoring devices help medical professionals tune treatments to an individual. Doctors are coaches as well as experts. People are more medically literate and collaborate in managing their healthcare, they monitor signals, intervene early and do not wait as long for illness to develop.

Private organisations (such as BUPA, Vitality, Nuffield Health and Echelon Health), tend to focus on medical factors. They carry out blood tests, look at indicators for heart, liver and kidney health, protein and muscle mass, and assess stroke risk. They may ignore other aspects of health and well-being. The fees that these organisations charge to carry out examinations put such testing out of the reach of many people, especially on a frequent basis.

In summary, the evidence supporting the significance of lifestyle factors in maintaining overall health seems clear and well founded. NHS waiting times have been increasing. People need to take care of themselves and in order to do that they need to be aware of their on-going health and wellbeing status. Yet, there are few tools or approaches available for them to evaluate and track a wide variety of aspects of their own (and dependents') health and wellbeing.

More From Life – How Are You?

One of the main drivers or catalysts for developing the *More From Life* approach was to combine a range of systemic tests and indicators of wellbeing, incorporated into one comprehensive, practical, inexpensive self-assessment tool. It is clear that changes in lifestyle and behaviour can produce rapid and dramatic improvements in many peoples' lives but there is little to help them achieve this.

Devices such as Fitbit and smart watches allow individuals to learn about certain quantifiable factors, such as steps per day and heart rate, but these provide a very limited view. Data presented in numerical, quantified form can be informative and useful. We need more of it, across a far broader variety of indicators.

Systems Thinking is a way of analysing complex situations by looking at context, relationships and interdependencies. It involves taking a holistic approach to problem-solving and decision-making, rather than focusing on individual components, as if these were isolated from the rest. A notional system can be imagined and described as a set of interconnected parts or sub-systems that work together. Changes in one part of a system have ripple effects throughout the entire system. Systems have inputs, outputs and processes. They are subject to change, including growth, adaptation and decay and are affected by their environment. A system can be viewed as being part of larger systems and have systems within it. The system as a whole is greater than the sum of its parts.

Humans can be thought of as complex systems. They have inputs, processes and outputs and are affected by their environment. They have interdependent, connected parts and subsystems that work together. They are part of larger systems. Changes to any part can have effects on the system as a whole. Humans are subject to change, growth and decay, (depending for example on many of the issues and factors discussed in this book).

More From Life uses system thinking concepts. It is the lifestyle, well-being and health awareness tool designed and developed to provide a wide-ranging and rich set of assessments. It prompts questions like "How fit, healthy and happy are you at the moment?" and "To what extent are you monitoring important indicators of your health and well-being?"

How healthy we are and how we feel depend on many different things, and we know that these things interact and affect each other. An important premise of *More From Life* is that paying attention to a variety of aspects of health and wellbeing tends to have beneficial effects in multiple ways which can boost each other. Consequently, *More From Life* is designed to help people to evaluate their present wellness status from many different perspectives, to let them to build a clearer picture. The idea is to offer tests, measurements and assessments to allow individuals to calculate scores for different aspects and indicators of their well-being.

A person's wellbeing changes over time, as they get older, experience changes in their circumstances, suffer from injury or illness and make changes to their lifestyle. *More From Life* can help them to track the impacts of these changes and see how they are doing. That said, these assessments are intended as indicators and awareness mechanisms, they do not constitute medical advice. This is not a medical textbook.

Cars have quite sophisticated monitoring systems that give you warnings of possible problems with the likes of: oil pressure, overheating, low fuel or water levels, and potential engine failure. We do not. We may not feel or learn about our own ill-health issues, that in many cases have been developing over a long time, until they become problematic and difficult to fix. Most of us do not have "engine" failure monitoring warnings. It would be so much better if warning lights flashed on our health and well-being dashboard before problems becomes more obvious, noticeable and serious.

While this book has been written with the assumption that you will want to work progressively through the chapters, take all the assessments and find out what your total *More From Life* score out of 500 is, some people may prefer to try just one or two of the sets of tests. For example, you may just want to take some of the exercise and fitness tests and / or answer the mental health questionnaires.

Chapter 3

MIND

How's life?

How happy are you?

Do you feel good? On top of the world or under the weather?

Are you content with the way things are?

The World Health Organization (WHO) defines mental health as "a state of well-being in which an individual realizes his or her own abilities, can cope with the normal stresses of life, can work productively and is able to make a contribution to his or her community".

In other words, mental health refers to the overall wellness of how we think, behave, act and look after our feelings. It includes our emotional, psychological, and social well-being. It controls how we see, interpret and react to things, the way we handle stress, relate to others, and make healthy choices. To a great extent, it determines our ability to enjoy life.

Mental Wellbeing self-assessment

Research shows that we need to take care of our mental health as well as our physical health. We should give ourselves time to relax and have fun, we should try to boost our happiness, engage with our friends and family, give and receive love, look after our work – life balance and have purpose in our lives. After all, the word "disease" comes from old French and means "lack of ease."

Numerous investigations have concluded that people who are lonely and depressed are 3 to 7 times more likely to become sick and die early. Research into the prevalence of major depressive and anxiety disorders due to the COVID-19 pandemic found that increases were associated with the combined effects of the spread of the virus, lockdowns, stay-at-home orders, school and business closures, and decreased social interactions, among other factors.

A study, published in the journal Nature, of phone calls to helplines in 19 countries, found that call volumes increased dramatically during the COVID pandemic. The NHS reported that the number of mental health calls to NHS 24 has risen 580% in four years and described the situation as a "mental health epidemic".

The number of antidepressant items prescribed in England increased by 34.8% in six years, from 61.9 million items in 2015/2016 to 83.4 million items in 2021/2022. Latest figures indicate that 8.32 million people, 14.7% of the population in England, received at least one prescription item for antidepressant drugs. Prescribing of antidepressants in children aged 5–12 years in the UK increased by more than 40% between 2015 and 2021.

The rapid increase in the use of opiates/opioids, such as morphine, heroin and fentanyl, since the 1990s in the US has had significant medical, social, psychological, and economic consequences. Despite the risk of abuse, addiction and overdose, the potency and availability of these substances have made them popular both as medical treatments and as recreational drugs. It is thought that 453,300 Americans died from opioid use between 1999 and 2016.

Approximately 1.5% of all deaths worldwide are by suicide (the act of intentionally causing one's own death), that is more than 700,000 deaths per year and it is estimated that there are 20 times as many attempts. Data published in 2019 by the WHO indicate that an average of 22.4 men and 6.8 women commit suicide per 100,000 population per year in the US, an increase of about 40% in 20 years. Mental disorders (including depression; schizophrenia; and bipolar, personality and anxiety disorders); substance abuse (including alcoholism and the use of and withdrawal from drugs); severe short and long term stress; employment and financial problems;

divorces and relationship difficulties; harassment and bullying are risk factors.

Our mental health affects the way we: interact, take care of ourself, take part in important activities, look after personal and family relationships, cope in social settings, learn, and get on at work or in education.

The following questionnaires aim to help you work out your current mental wellbeing score. The questions are designed to help you to assess your feelings and state of mind. They are based on recognised assessments such as WEMWBS (Warwick-Edinburgh Mental Well-being Scale), WHO, HADS (the Hospital Anxiety and Depression Scale) and PANAS (the Positive and Negative Affect Schedule).

The questions are organised into four sections or groups:

- How relaxed or stressed you've been
- Your happiness and how you feel about yourself
- Your work / life balance
- Your relationships and personal life

To obtain your up-to-date wellbeing scores go through the following questions and circle the number (from 0 to 10) that is closest to your thoughts and feelings about each issue or question over the last few days. For example, if you feel really calm and relaxed all the time circle 10 in question 1. Try not to overthink this assessment – just go with your feelings.

1) Relaxation and Stress

Section A

1 - I feel relaxed and calm										
Never										Always
0	1	2	3	4	5	6	7	8	9	10

2 - I have been thinking clearly and can concentrate										
Never										Always
0	1	2	3	4	5	6	7	8	9	10

3 - I have plenty of chances to catch up with things I need to do										
Never										Always
0	1	2	3	4	5	6	7	8	9	10

4 - I take time out to read, listen to music, or go for a walk										
Never										Often
0	1	2	3	4	5	6	7	8	9	10

5 - I practice Meditation and / or Mindfulness										
Never										Often
0	1	2	3	4	5	6	7	8	9	10

6 - I like where I live, and I feel safe and secure										
Never										Often
0	1	2	3	4	5	6	7	8	9	10

Section B

7 - I feel tired and have little energy										
Always										Never
0	1	2	3	4	5	6	7	8	9	10

8 - I become upset, distressed or nervous easily										
Often										Never
0	1	2	3	4	5	6	7	8	9	10

9 - I experience sudden mood swings and unexpected waves of anxiety and panic										
Often										Never
0	1	2	3	4	5	6	7	8	9	10

10 - I am tense, restless, agitated and on edge										
Always										Never
0	1	2	3	4	5	6	7	8	9	10

Score = (/100)

2) Happiness and Self-esteem

Section A

1 - I feel that life is very good, I am happy										
Never										Always
0	1	2	3	4	5	6	7	8	9	10

2 - I tend to laugh and see the funny side of things										
Never										Always
0	1	2	3	4	5	6	7	8	9	10

3 - I have fun										
Never										Always
0	1	2	3	4	5	6	7	8	9	10

4 - I feel strong, proud, confident and good about myself										
Never										Always
0	1	2	3	4	5	6	7	8	9	10

5 - I've been feeling optimistic about the future and look forward to things										
Never										Always
0	1	2	3	4	5	6	7	8	9	10

6 - I care about my appearance										
Never										Always
0	1	2	3	4	5	6	7	8	9	10

Section B

7 - I have little interest in, or pleasure doing, things.										
Always										Never
0	1	2	3	4	5	6	7	8	9	10

8 - I feel down, depressed, lonely or hopeless.										
Always										Never
0	1	2	3	4	5	6	7	8	9	10

9 - I am worried about some of my habits and behaviour, (eg alcohol, drugs, gambling, anger).										
Always										Never
0	1	2	3	4	5	6	7	8	9	10

10 - I worry and get anxious about what people say about me.										
Always										Never
0	1	2	3	4	5	6	7	8	9	10

Score = (/100)

3) Work-life Balance

Section A

1 - I feel useful, needed and appreciated										
Never										Always
0	1	2	3	4	5	6	7	8	9	10

2 - I enjoy challenges and deal with problems well										
Never										Always
0	1	2	3	4	5	6	7	8	9	10

3 - I find it easy to manage all my duties and responsibilities										
Never										Always
0	1	2	3	4	5	6	7	8	9	10

4 I feel financially secure										
Never										Always
0	1	2	3	4	5	6	7	8	9	10

5 I've been able to make up my own mind about things										
Never										Always
0	1	2	3	4	5	6	7	8	9	10

Section B

6 - I am bullied										
Always										Never
0	1	2	3	4	5	6	7	8	9	10

7 - I ignore and neglect some important things										
Always										Never
0	1	2	3	4	5	6	7	8	9	10

8 - I feel bad about myself, as if I am a bit of a failure and have let people down										
Always										Never
0	1	2	3	4	5	6	7	8	9	10

9 - I feel burnt-out and worried about the way things are going										
Always										Never
0	1	2	3	4	5	6	7	8	9	10

10 - I feel as though there is not enough time in the day										
Always										Never
0	1	2	3	4	5	6	7	8	9	10

Score = (/100)

4) Relationships and Personal Life

Section A

1 - I feel loved.										
Never										Always
0	1	2	3	4	5	6	7	8	9	10

2 - People take an interest in what I say and do.										
Never										Always
0	1	2	3	4	5	6	7	8	9	10

3 - I have an active social life.										
Never										Always
0	1	2	3	4	5	6	7	8	9	10

4 - I enjoy being with, and looking after, pets.										
Never										Always
0	1	2	3	4	5	6	7	8	9	10

5 - I appreciate and enjoy life, I get out and "smell the flowers".										
Never										Always
0	1	2	3	4	5	6	7	8	9	10

6 - I make an effort to have a cheerful and positive effect on others.										
Never										Always
0	1	2	3	4	5	6	7	8	9	10

Section B

7 - I am experiencing difficult challenges, eg bereavement, changing job, moving house, marriage, children, ...											
Often											Never
0	1	2	3	4	5	6	7	8	9	10	

8 - When things get difficult, I have no one to turn to. My friends disappear.											
Often											Never
0	1	2	3	4	5	6	7	8	9	10	

9 - People think or say that I seem irritable, angry and or hostile.											
Often											Never
0	1	2	3	4	5	6	7	8	9	10	

10 - There is friction, tension and unpleasantness between my family/ friends / colleagues											
Often											Never
0	1	2	3	4	5	6	7	8	9	10	

Score = (/100)

Now add all 4 scores to give you a total out of 400 and then divide by 4.

Total score for the Mind section = (/100).

Mental health is important at every stage of life. Sometimes people experience significant disturbances and distress that disrupt their ability to function or feel happy. Mental health can include feelings of anger, hopelessness, depression, loneliness, stress, anxiety, sleep problems, phobias, hoarding, panic attacks, drug and alcohol addiction, paranoia, self-esteem, voices, eating problems, post-traumatic stress disorder and suicidal feelings. If you find that you have given yourself very low marks and you feel depressed you should consider contacting your doctor or a health professional. Ask for help if you feel suicidal.

Ten Strategies to Improve How You Feel

Research suggests there are several ways we can improve our mental health and wellbeing.

1. Be active physically. Do lots of walking, ideally outdoors in the countryside, through a forest, in hills and ancient woodlands, or barefoot on a beach. Better still go with friends and a dog or two. Try a long cut through a park. Take long strides or walk more quickly than usual, raise your heart rate a bit. Evidence shows this helps us to feel better, it changes our mood and makes us feel more positive. If you haven't already, try jogging or running. The "Couch to 5Km program is a great way to start and "Parkrun"s happen every week in most cities. Take up or try other sports such as swimming, ice skating, horse riding, cycling or better still participate in sports that involve other people such as 5-a-side football, badminton, frisbee, softball, tennis, basketball and hockey.

2. Improve connections with other people. Make friends and join up with new groups. Good relationships are often fundamental for our mental wellbeing. They help our sense of belonging and self-worth, give us opportunities to share experiences, provide us with emotional support and allow us to support others. There are many ways to build stronger and closer relationships: try to connect with friends and family as often as possible, arrange meals for example so that you can all eat at the same time together, instead of spending time on social media or watching TV, use video chat more often, have days out or play games with friends, family and children. Visit people who need support or company. Volunteer at a local charity, hospital or community group.

3. Breathing exercises can help to us to stay calm and reduce feelings of stress and panic. They can be done anywhere and at almost any time. Begin by making yourself comfortable, if you're lying down, place your arms a little bit away from your sides, with the palms up, and bend your knees so your feet are flat on the floor. Breathe in gently, feel it expand your chest and stomach. Some people find it helpful to count steadily from 1 to 5. Then let your breath flow out gently, counting from 1 to 5 again. Spend at least 5 minutes taking quite deep regular breaths, in through your nose and out through your mouth.

4. Taking up a new sport or hobby or learning new skills can help to boost our self-confidence, give us more of a sense of purpose, and develop relationships with others. Ideas include learning: to play the guitar or piano, a new language, new cooking skills, gardening and growing plants and vegetables, becoming better at photography, drawing and painting, trying Geocaching, writing a blog, making videos, studying and practicing DIY. Make an effort to change your routine and habits.

5. Be kind and thoughtful. Research suggests that offering support and friendship, giving help and gifts, doing favours, asking people how they are and listening to their answers, and performing acts of kindness can make us feel better. We not only feel more positive and useful but also communicate better with others.

6. Pay attention to the present moment. Mindfulness can help us to enjoy life more as we gain a better understanding of ourself, become more aware of aspects we often ignore or miss (such as birdsong, flowers, clouds and sunsets), and appreciate the world around us. Don't take things for granted. It is said that by paying more attention to the present moment, our thoughts and feelings, our body and environment, we can improve our wellbeing.

7. Listen to music and, if you like, sing along or dance. Research evidence suggests that music can lift our mood, reduce our stress and anxiety, lower our blood pressure, relieve symptoms of depression, ease and manage pain, boost our immune system, increase our motivation, enhance our performance, improve our sleep, regulate our nervous system, and stimulate our creativity, problem solving and memory. Furthermore, we often feel much happier when we sing and dance.

8. Analyse and take control of the situation. One of the main causes of stress for many people is feeling that they are losing control. This can feel similar to the fight or flight impulse, we are trapped. Taking more control is, in itself, empowering, and an important part of finding a solution that is satisfactory to us and others. Talking things through with a friend can empower and help us to review options and find answers to problems.

9. Be positive and accept the things we cannot change. We cannot please all the people all the time. It is not always possible to improve or resolve difficult situations. We should concentrate on the things we can do something about. Look for the positives in life, the aspects and things we are grateful for. Write them down in a journal every day if that helps. Organise and prioritise a to do list, what needs to be done, your tasks and work, allow yourself some "me" time and get sufficient sleep.

10. Avoid unhealthy habits. Do not rely on drugs, alcohol and smoking as short-term friends for happiness or as ways of coping. They may provide temporary relief, but in the long run, these crutches often make our problems worse.

Chapter 4

BODY

What do you know?

We all want to stay healthy for as long as possible, but do you know if your body is in good condition?

- Is it running like a trusted, well-maintained machine or breaking down?
- Is it showing signs of illness such as CVD or diabetes or hypertension or inflammation?
- Are you functioning properly or feeling the effects of age, wear and tear?
- How are your guts, organs, skin and senses?
- What can we do to monitor our body's health?
- What should we be testing and tracking?
- What aspects of us are ok and what may need attention and or help?

There are several assessments you can try yourself to check and measure different aspects of your medical health. The Body quarter of the *More From Life* circle helps you to evaluate some important indicators and biomarkers. It should be emphasised that these basic DIY tests may not produce results that are as accurate as those provided by laboratory tests. If you are concerned about any of the findings or results you should get them checked by your doctor – this book only suggests some basic tests, some of which may be unreliable, it does not give medical advice.

First let's take some measurements (mostly in centimetres):

Type	Measurement	
	Initial	After challenges
Height:		
Waist:		
Chest:		
Hips:		
Biceps:		
Thighs:		
Weight (in Kilograms):		
Today's Date:		

1) Twenty starter questions

We begin the Body assessments with 20 background questions about aspects of your overall health, split into 3 parts.

Section A

Award yourself 1 point for every time you answer YES to the following 5 questions.	Yes or No?
Have you had a dental check-up within the last 12 months?	
Have you been for an eyesight test within the last 12 months?	
Are you reasonably full of energy and get up and go? Can you keep going all day?	
Would you say that you can breathe easily through your nose?	
Have you checked your skin* within the last month?	

*You should keep an eye on and know about your skin spots and moles so that you can notice potentially dangerous problems and diseases like skin cancer. Skin cancer is a common form of cancer but it is almost always treatable when caught early. Observant patients and their partners are more likely to see melanomas before their doctors, especially if they know what to look for.

Scan your entire body, beginning with your face and working downward, checking your neck, shoulders, chest, arms (front, back, and sides) and legs (front, back, and sides). Don't forget your groin, palms, fingernails, soles of your feet, toenails, and the areas between your toes. Take photos of any parts you cannot see. The ABCDE (which stands for Asymmetry, Border, Colour, Diameter, and Evolving) method is a good way to help you check yourself. If any moles look misshapen / Asymmetrical or have an irregular or poorly defined Border or if the Colour is not consistent but varies, or if the Diameter is greater than 6 millimetres (the size of the end of a pencil) or the mole is Evolving in shape and size, have it checked by a dermatologist or medical professional.

Section B

Give yourself 1 point every time you answer NO to one of the following 5 questions.	Yes or No?
Do you sometimes have chest pains?	
Do not have a persistent cough?	
Have you noticed any abnormal bleeding?	
Have you been suffering from severe or frequent headaches recently?	
Do you feel out of breath when you climb a flight of stairs?	

If you have experienced chest pains recently or had a persistent cough for 3 weeks or more or you suspect or have seen evidence of unusual blood or bleeding or you feel breathless climbing a flight of stairs or you have experienced a sudden increase in headaches or pain it may be worthwhile discussing this with a doctor.

Section C

During the last few days, ...	Yes or No?
Have you had bad pain in your tummy or abdomen?	
Have you had strange, unusual pain anywhere else?	
Have you felt dizzy or faint?	
Have you lost your appetite or sense of smell?	
Have you been feeling unusually tired and fatigued?	
Have you been feeling bloated?	
Have you been vomiting?	
Have you been feverish / had a high temperature?	
Have you felt unusually cold / shivering?	
Do you have swollen ankles, feet or legs (oedema)?	
Give yourself 1 point every time you answered NO Total	

If you answered YES to any of these questions it is important to say that, while many of these symptoms and indications may be routine and nothing to worry about, they can sometimes signal issues that need consideration and attention.

Total points for question 1 = (/20)

2) Resting Heart Rate

Studies have shown that a lower resting heart rate is often associated with a longer life span. For every 20 additional beats per minute (bpm) of resting heart rate, mortality increases by 30 to 50 percent. The association between a low resting heart rate and lifespan appears to work through at least two distinct mechanisms. Firstly, a slower heart rate is associated with a healthier heart, people with a low resting heart rate are far less likely to die of cardiac illness. Secondly, a slower heart rate is associated with a slower metabolic rate. Slower metabolism can mean that, in effect, everything is slowed down, you are less active and may be more prone to weight gain if you overeat, but since your body is running more slowly, it may age more slowly.

In a few cases a resting heart rate below 60bpm may cause dizziness, fatigue, sweating, or fainting and be called bradycardia, if you have these symptoms, it is worth discussing things with your doctor.

Instructions: if you wear a smart watch, observe your resting heart rate at times when you are relaxed and inactive. If you do not have a smart watch press your fingertips lightly on the inside of your wrist (where the buckle of a watch might be) and find the beating pulse. Take a watch with a second hand or a stop watch and sit quietly for a few moments. When you feel calm and relaxed, count the number of pulses / beats that occur in a minute.

Resting Heart Rate (HR) – beats per minute					
HR	<60	61 - 70	71 - 80	81 - 90	91 - 100	>100
Points	5	4	3	2	1	0

Score for Resting Heart Rate test = (/5)

3) Reaction Time Test

Reaction time (RT) is a measure of the quickness with which an organism responds to some sort of stimulus. RT is defined as the interval of time between the presentation of the stimulus and appearance of appropriate voluntary response in the subject. Reaction time is important in our everyday lives, it is an indicator of a healthy functioning sensory system, cognitive processing and motor performance. Reaction times relate to a person's coordination and performance. A good reaction time allows us to be more agile and efficient when it comes to responding to stimuli in situations like driving, playing sports, and having a conversation.

This assessment is worth 5 points. It has two options; a) and b), you can do one or the other. Option a) invites you to take an on-line test, option b) invites you to try the Ruler reaction time test.

a) There are apps and tools on-line that are easy to use, (such as Human Benchmark and the online reaction time test at Washington.edu).

Instructions: Go to the humanbenchmark.com website and click on the "Reaction Time" box. When you click on the large blue space at the top of the next screen, it will turn red. Click again as soon as it turns green and your reaction time will be displayed (in milliseconds) You can try this test as many times as you like.

On-Line Reaction Time Test (RT) – (number of milliseconds)						
RT	<150	151 - 200	201 - 250	251 - 300	301 - 399	>400
Points	5	4	3	2	1	0

b) Alternatively, if you do not have access to the website, you can try the Ruler Reaction Time test. All you need is an ordinary ruler and someone's help.

Instructions: Sit in a chair with one of your forearms (from elbow to wrist) resting on a table or arm rest, so that only your hand protrudes beyond the table or arm rest. Turn your hand so that it is in the same position that it would be to hold a glass of water, with your thumb and fingers about 2 centimetres apart. You are going to catch (trap between your thumb and finger tips) a ruler as it falls.

When you are ready, ask the other person to hold the ruler vertically just above your thumb and fingers (so that the lowest part of the ruler is just above the top of your hand). They are going to let it go without warning. Wait for them to release and let the ruler drop and catch it as soon as you can. Measure how far the ruler descended, before you caught it, by looking at the point on the ruler just above your thumb. Use the table to work out your score. For example if you caught the ruler after it had descended 12 centimetres, you score 3 points.

You can have 5 attempts at this test.

Ruler Reaction Time Test						
Ruler (cms)	Dropped	>25	<20	<15	<10	<5
Points	0	1	2	3	4	5

Score for Reaction Time test = (/5)

4) Brain / Memory test

This experiment will test your thinking and memory and can be run multiple times. You need a pack of ordinary playing cards and a stop watch. You are going to look for pairs of cards.

Instructions: Place all 52 cards face down on the floor, spread them out so that they do not touch each other. It might be easier to lay them out in 4 or 5 or 6 rows. Start the stop watch. Turn the first 2 cards over (face up) look at them, then turn them back face down and pick up two more, continue like this, trying to remember where each card is. When you get a pair (for example you overturn 2 kings at the same time) remove these two cards from the floor. Keep going until you have paired and removed all the cards. How long did it take to clear the floor of cards? Compare your time to the table below and give yourself a score out of 10.

Brain / Memory Test	
Minutes	Points
Less than 3:00	10
3:01 to 3:30	9
3:31 to 4:00	8
4:00 to 4:30	7
4:31 to 5:00	6
5:01 to 5:30	5
5:31 to 6:00	4
6:01 to 6:30	3
6:31 to 7:00	2
7:01 to 8:00	1
Over 8 minutes	0

Score for Brain / Memory test = (/10)

Composition

Body fat (or adipose tissue) secretes a number of important hormones and stores lipids from which the body creates energy and provides us with some cushioning and insulation.

Some types of body fat can have negative effects on us, others are beneficial and necessary for our health. The main types are white, brown, and beige cells. They can be stored as essential, subcutaneous, or visceral fat.

- White fat is the large, white cells that are stored under the skin or around the organs in the tummy, buttocks, arms and thighs. These fat cells are the body's way of storing energy for later use. White fat plays a role in the function of hormones but too much white fat is harmful.

- Brown fat is found in babies, although adults do retain a small amount, typically in the neck and shoulders. It helps to keep you warm and researchers are interested in finding ways to stimulate the activity of brown fat to prevent obesity.

- Beige fat is believed to function somewhere between brown and white fat cells. Like brown fat, beige cells help to burn fat rather than store it. Certain hormones and enzymes that are released when we are stressed, do exercise or get cold are thought to convert white fat into beige fat.

- Essential fat is essential for a healthy body. It is found in our: nerves, brain, bone marrow and the membranes that protect our organs. Essential fat plays an important role in controlling fertility, vitamin absorption, and temperature regulation.

- Subcutaneous is the layer of fat under our skin. It insulates and protects our body.

- Visceral fat, also known as "spare tyre belly fat," is the white fat which is stored in our abdomen and surrounds our major organs, (our liver, kidneys, pancreas, intestines, and heart). Having high levels of visceral fat is known to increase our risk of getting diabetes, heart disease, stroke, artery disease, and some cancers.

Women and men store body fat differently and this can change over time. The amount of essential fat for men is around 2-5% and 10-13% in women. The healthy range of body fat for men is usually defined as 8-19%, while the healthy range for women is 21-33%.

Excess body fat can have many detrimental effects on a person's health, but insufficient body fat can also have negative health effects. Excess body fat leads to being overweight and eventually to obesity. Managing diet and exercise has been shown to reduce stored fat. The World Health Organization (WHO) classifies obesity as one of the leading preventable causes of death worldwide. Obesity is associated with a reduction in quality of life, poorer mental health outcomes, obstructive sleep apnoea, increases in "bad" cholesterol, as well as cardiovascular disease, stroke, certain cancers and diabetes. All of these potential complications can and do reduce a person's life expectancy.

5) BMI (Body Mass Index)

A well-known and commonly used way to judge whether someone is overweight or obese is by comparing their height to their weight in a calculation named the BMI formula (kg/m2).

This assessment has been criticised. Critics say that BMI is not always a good indicator of percent of body fat and that BMI may not be as accurate or useful as some other measurements. Using BMI as a guide, people who have lots of muscle may seem overweight yet be healthy. Muscle has more density than fat. Rugby players, for example, although fit and healthy may have high BMI measurements. For these reasons BMI is only awarded 5 *More From Life* points.

Instructions: *Divide your weight in kilograms by your height in metres, then divide that answer by your height. That's your BMI!*

For example: If a person weighs 70kg and they are 1.75m tall, we divide their weight (70) by their height (1.75), = 40. Then divide that (40) by their height, which comes to a BMI score of 22.857.

	BMI measurement					
BMI	<18	18 to 22	23 to 25	26 to 30	31 to 40	>40
Points	3	5	4	3	1	0

Score for BMI test = (/5)

Body fat and waist circumference measurements are probably more useful ways to look at the big picture of overall health, determine potential disease risk and the chances of developing serious conditions like diabetes, stroke, sleep apnoea, and heart disease. Body fat and waist circumference are indicators of the fat that often surrounds internal organs and is regarded as the most dangerous. We should keep our waist circumference to less than half our height.

6) Waist to Height Ratio calculation

The Waist to Height ratio focuses on the part of the body that is likely to exhibit visceral fat.

Instructions: *Measure your waist circumference at a horizontal line one inch above your belly button. Ratio = Waist measurement (in centimetres) divided by your Height (in centimetres). Circle your result in the table below:*

Waist to Height Ratio			
Women	Men	Points	
<0.35	<0.35	6	Very Slim
0.35 to 0.41	0.35 to 0.41	8	Slim
	0.42 to 0.43	9	Marginal
0.42 to 0.48	0.44 to 0.5	10	Healthy
	0.51 to 0.52	9	Marginal
0.49 to 0.5	0.53 to 0.54	8	
0.51 to 0.52	0.55 to 0.56	7	Overweight
0.53 to 0.54	0.57 to 0.57	6	
0.55 to 0.56	0.58 to 0.59	5	Very Overweight
0.57	0.6 to 0.61	4	
0.58	0.62 to 0.63	3	
0.59	0.64 to 0.65	2	
0.6 to 0.63	0.66 to 0.69	1	Obese
> 0.63	>0.7	0	

Score for Waist to Height Ratio assessment = (/10)

7) Body Fat

Bioelectrical impedance analysis is a way of determining body fat percentage. It is often used in athletic training facilities. Many modern digital bathroom scales claim to measure weight, body fat, muscle mass, bone mass, body water, visceral fat, subcutaneous fat, protein mass, and obesity level.

Instructions: *The test involves standing on, or holding, a device (such as modern weighing machine or a handheld body fat analyser) that uses electrical current to measure the amount of lean versus fatty mass in your body. Follow the instructions offered by the device.*

Body Fat Measurement							
Men	<5	<15	<20	<25	<30	<35	>35
Women	<10	<20	<25	<30	<35	<40	>40
Points	2	5	4	3	2	1	0

Score for Body Fat measurement = (/5)

8) Blood Pressure

Your *Blood Pressure* is another measurement everyone should pay attention to in order to assess and maintain their overall health. Blood pressure is the force that our blood exerts on the walls of our arteries. It is measured as two numbers – the systolic and the diastolic pressures. These are usually described as the systolic over the diastolic (for example 120 over 80). High blood pressure (Hypertension) is known as the "silent killer" because it may not have obvious symptoms but it can contribute to the damage of important vessels in your body and increase the risk of heart attack or stroke.

Hypertension affects about 1 in 3 adults in the UK and unhealthy lifestyles are known to be the main cause. To reduce your blood pressure you need to: maintain a healthy weight, exercise regularly, relax more, sleep well, eat foods rich in potassium, avoid tobacco and processed food and limit consumption of salt, sugar, alcohol and saturated fat.

Instructions: do not: drink coffee or alcohol, or smoke, or do exercise, or eat, or take medication for about 30 minutes before starting this test. Find a comfortable chair, sit down, rest your feet on the floor and your arm on an arm rest and relax for 5 minutes. Follow the instructions that came with the monitor. Place the correct size of inflatable arm cuff just above your elbow, preferably on bare skin, about the same height as your heart. Stay still and try not to talk while the device inflates, deflates and takes your reading. Take two or three readings, each a few minutes apart. You can do this several times a day and observe the differences.

Blood Pressure assessment table

		Points						
Systolic	190+	0	0	0	0	0	0	0
	180	0	0	0	0	0	0	0
	170	1	1	1	1	1	1	1
	160	3	3	3	3	3	2	1
	150	4	4	4	4	4	2	1
	140	5	5	5	5	5	5	1
	130	7	7	7	7	7	6	1
	120	10	10	10	10	9	6	2
	110	10	10	10	10	9	6	2
	100	10	10	10	10	9	6	2
	90	9		10	10	9	6	2
	80	7		10	10	9	6	2
	70	4		10	10	9	6	2
		40	50	60	70	80	90	100
		Diastolic						

Score for Blood Pressure measurement = (/10)

9) Cholesterol

Cholesterol is a type of fat or lipid that is carried around the body in the blood. Eating fatty food, not exercising enough, being overweight, smoking and drinking alcohol increase your chances of having higher cholesterol levels which can build up as deposits in your arteries and increase your risk of heart attack or stroke. Although a high level of cholesterol is often a significant risk factor for coronary artery disease, it may not cause any symptoms, so you could have it without knowing. For that reason, a cholesterol test is an important tool. It can help to determine your risk of the build-up of fatty deposits (plaques) in your blood vessels that can lead to narrowed or blocked arteries throughout your body (atherosclerosis). Please note that this is just one of the cholesterol assessments – you should keep an eye on your Apolipoprotein B (ApoB), HDL, LDL, triglycerides and cholesterol ratio as well.

Instructions: to use a cholesterol home test kit, follow the instructions that come with the product. Typically, you will be asked to prick your finger with a lancet, then place a blood droplet on the test strip. The cholesterol home test strip has special chemicals that change colours after a few minutes. You match the final colour against a colour guide that's included with the kit. You are generally required to fast beforehand, - consuming no food or liquids other than water, for 9 to 12 hours before the test, however some cholesterol tests do not require fasting. Some, usually more expensive, cholesterol home test kits have an electronic meter. The test strips are inserted into the electronic device and a small computer measures the amount of cholesterol automatically. Consult the table of cholesterol test values and award yourself points out of 10, for example if your test produced a value of 4.8 give yourself 6 points.

Cholesterol test	
Level	Points
<3.4	10
<3.8	9
<4.2	8
<4.6	7
<5	6
<5.4	5
<5.8	4
<6.2	3
<6.6	2
<7	1
>7	0

Score for Cholesterol test =   (out of 10)

10) Blood sugar

Your blood sugar level usually rises when you eat. Your cells can take that sugar out of the bloodstream and use it for energy, but only with the help of insulin, a hormone made by the pancreas. When you have diabetes, your body does not make enough insulin or does not use it effectively, and too much sugar is left in your blood. Over time, this can damage your circulation, eyes, kidneys, nerves, and heart so you should measure the amount of glucose in your blood regularly.

Many people who discover that they have diabetes report that they had no signs or warnings of the disease. Symptoms include: increased hunger and thirst; increased urination, particularly at night; unexplained weight loss; unexplainable tiredness; blurred vision; high blood pressure, slow-healing sores or wounds that appear to heal and then reopen. However, lack of symptoms does not necessarily mean the absence of diabetes.

Diabetes is the seventh leading cause of death in the United States. The disease can lead to many complications, including: stroke, heart attack, and blood clots; wounds, numbness, tingling; amputation of feet or limbs; kidney failure; nerve damage; chronic headaches; vision and hearing loss. Blindness can occur overnight. Early interventions and regular glucose monitoring reduce the risk of severe or potentially fatal diabetes complications.

Studies going back over 50 years have found that people who eat meat, (even just one day a week), have significantly higher rates of diabetes and the more frequently they ate meat, the more frequently the disease occurred. Those eating plant-based diets had a fraction of the diabetes rates, they have improved reductions in blood sugars, body weight, and cardio vascular risk factors compared to people who consume animal products. What is more, with a plant-based diet, there is less need to worry about calorie counting.

Instructions: *follow the guidelines that come with the pack. Home blood glucose tests are safe and affordable, they usually include glucose testing strips that a machine uses to detect the level of glucose in a drop of blood.*

Blood Glucose test		
Levels	Points	Notes
<3	3	Low
<4	9	Normal
<5	8	
<6	7	
<7	4	Pre-diabetic
<8	3	Diabetic Consult doctor
<9	2	
<10	1	
<11	0	High risk
>11	0	Seek medical help

Score for Blood Sugar level measurement = (/10)

CGM or flash monitors, such as the FreeStyle Libre BP meter, are said not to require finger-prick blood samples. Instead, these meters read glucose from interstitial fluids just underneath the skin. The Freestyle works via a sensor you wear on the back of your upper arm, which you apply every 14 days.

11) Poo / Faeces / Stools

Poo is what is left of what you consume after your body absorbs important nutrients. It is the waste products that the body eliminates, including: undigested food particles, bacteria, salts, and other substances. Your bowel habits are a strong indicator of your digestive health. Changes in the colour, shape and texture of your stool can reveal signs of infection, digestive issues or more serious health problems.

Causes of constipation, diarrhoea, and other poo abnormalities include: dehydration, stress, depression, inactivity, lack of dietary fibre, allergies, IBS, cancer, Parkinson's, and an overactive or underactive thyroid. You should contact a doctor if changes to your poo persist for 2 weeks or more. Seek immediate medical advice if your poo is bright red, black, or tarry, these signs may suggest blood loss, which could become a medical emergency if left untreated.

Instructions: observe your poos and note their colour, consistency, unusual characteristics and frequency. Using the table below select the most appropriate description and corresponding points.

Poo / Faeces / Stools	
Description	Points
Long, brown, snake or hot-dog, sausage shaped poos that are comfortable and easy to pass.	5
A bit too hard or firm or too soft / fluffy or mushy, can be caused by a lack of fibre.	4
Greasy yellow usually means you are eating too much fat.	3
Pale or white or cream coloured may mean the poo lacks bile and could be a sign you need to talk to a health professional	2
Chronic diarrhoea (completely watery with few if any solids and maybe more than 5 times a day) or Chronic constipation (less than 3 times a week, hard marble-like pellets that may take 15 minutes or more to pass). If these persist for a few days without explanation consult a doctor.	1
Possible danger signs = painful or with mucus or silver or red or black and tarry (these colours may be due to something you ate like beetroot or liquorice or iron supplements, if not it might be blood, consult a doctor immediately).	0

Score for Faeces / Poo = (/5)

12) Pulse Oximeter / Blood Oxygen

We need a constant supply of oxygen to survive. Our lungs transmit oxygen, through tiny capillary blood vessels, to the heart, which pumps it to the rest of the body. SpO_2 measurement or pulse oximetry is a painless method of assessing the saturation of oxygen in our blood which is a good way to measure how well our breathing and lungs are working. A pulse oximeter is a small, electronic device which can be clipped onto a fingertip. It emits light that passes through the fingernail, skin, tissue, and blood. A sensor, on the other side of the finger, detects and measures the amount of light that passes through without getting absorbed by the tissue and blood and, from that, the device estimates the oxygen saturation of the blood. Some of the cheaper SpO_2 meters can be 2% or 3% inaccurate. Nail varnish and false nails can block the light and affect the reading.

Lower oxygen saturation levels may be caused by: an asthma attack, scarred and damaged lungs, pneumonia, COVID-19, fluid or blood clot in the lungs, collapsed lung, cardiovascular diseases, anaemia, sleep apnoea, acute respiratory distress syndrome (ARDS), chronic obstructive pulmonary diseases (COPD) including emphysema and chronic bronchitis, certain pain medications and other drugs that can weaken breathing, such as narcotics, anaesthetics and poisoning.

The pulse oximeter test can be done while seated at home as an occasional measurement or it can be used to measure your oxygen levels over a period of time, for example during exercise like walking or when you are asleep.

A resting oxygen saturation level between 95% and 100% is regarded as normal for a healthy person at sea level. At higher elevations, oxygen saturation levels may be slightly lower. People should contact a health care provider if their oxygen saturation readings persistently drop below 92%, as it may be a sign of hypoxia, a serious condition in which not enough oxygen reaches the body's organs and tissues. If blood oxygen saturation levels fall to 88% or lower, consider seeking immediate medical attention.

Instructions: *place the pulse oximeter over your fingertip and note the reading.*

Pulse Oximeter / SpO$_2$ meter	
Ranges (%)	Points
98 to 100	5
96 to 98	4
93 to 95	3
91 to 92	2
89 to 90	1
Less than 89	0

Score for Blood Oxygen level = (/5)

Total score for the Body section = (/100).

Other Considerations

There are of course other aspects of health that you should keep track of, such as your eyes, mouth, teeth and skin. For example: normal vision shouldn't be blurred, have black spots or double vision, the whites of the eyes should not be yellow (which could indicate jaundice) or red (possible infection or inflammation) and any changes may require medical investigation. An eye condition called Age-related Macular Degeneration (AMD) is the most common cause of loss of sight in the UK and the leading cause of blindness for people over 50. To test for it look at a door frame or large window frame from across a room with one eye and then the other by putting your palm over an eye for 30 seconds. If you see a bend or crookedness in the frame's straight line it can be a sign of AMD.

Chapter 5

EXERCISE

Would you like to feel better, have more energy and add years to your active life?

Then you need to exercise.

The benefits of regular exercise and physical activity are proven and hard to ignore. There is irrefutable evidence of the effectiveness of regular physical activity in the treatment and prevention of several chronic diseases including: type 2 diabetes, cardio vascular disease, cancer, hypertension, obesity and depression.

Everyone benefits from exercise no matter what age, gender or physical ability. It adds years to your life and life to your years.

Physical inactivity has been called one of the biggest public health problems of the 21st century. Many of us are too sedentary. Not walking for about an hour a day is considered a high-risk behaviour. These days, doctors are encouraged to prescribe exercise and walking. Exercise has been found to work as well as drugs in some cases, especially when combined with improvements in diet.

Eight benefits of exercise:

- *Exercise helps you to control your weight and the fat / muscle ratio* – exercise can be part of a strategy to prevent excess weight gain and maintain weight loss. When you engage in physical activity you burn calories. The more intense the activity the more calories you burn. Vigorous exercise can raise your metabolic rate so you carry on burning calories long after the exercise. Sweating helps to eliminate toxins.

- *Exercise combats many health conditions and diseases* – it helps lower the risk of death from all causes. Regular exercise helps prevent or manage a wide range of health problems and concerns, including stroke, metabolic syndrome, high blood pressure, type 2 diabetes, stress, depression, anxiety, many types of cancer, arthritis, skin problems and falls. It can also help to improve memory and cognitive function.

- *Exercise improves mood* – *a* gym session or brisk walk can help lift you mentally. Physical activity stimulates various brain chemicals that can leave you feeling happier, more relaxed and less anxious. Dopamine, Serotonin, Oxytocin and Endorphins are "happy hormones" that play key roles in our mood, sleep, digestion, nausea, wound healing, pain relief, bone health, blood clotting and sexual desire. You may also feel better about your appearance and yourself when you exercise regularly, which can boost your confidence and enhance your self-esteem.

- *Exercise boosts strength, resilience, endurance* and flexibility - regular physical activity can improve your strength, reduce muscle wastage, make you more flexible and less prone to injury and improve your stamina and endurance. Research reveals that strength training improves the mineral density of the bones, protecting you from osteoporosis. Strength training also helps improve muscle mass, muscle power, and muscle endurance.

- *Exercise gives you more energy* – it delivers oxygen and nutrients to your tissues and helps your cardiovascular system work more efficiently and effectively. You have more energy to tackle daily life when your heart and lung health improves.

- *Exercise promotes better sleep* - physical activity helps you fall asleep faster and have better, deeper, more restorative sleep. Your muscles, bones, and brain are rejuvenated while you sleep.

- *Exercise can invigorate, freshen and put the sparkle back into your sex life* - do you feel too tired or too out of shape to enjoy physical intimacy? Regular physical activity can improve testosterone, energy levels and physical appearance and boost your sex life. Regular physical activity may enhance arousal for women, and men who exercise regularly are less likely to have problems with erectile dysfunction than men who do not exercise.

- *Exercise can be sociable and enjoyable fun* - physical activity gives you a chance to unwind, enjoy the outdoors, engage in activities that make you happy and team up with other people. Physical activities can help you connect in social settings.

Physical Activity

Regular physical activity is a good way to stay fit, feel better, boost your health and have fun. We should try to be active most of the day, staying on our feet and moving around as much as possible. At least 150 minutes a week of moderate aerobic activity or 75 minutes a week of vigorous aerobic activity a week, (or a combination of moderate and vigorous activity) is recommended for most reasonably healthy adults. Examples include walking, dancing, running or swimming. We should fit in strength training for all the major muscle groups, at least twice a week, by lifting free weights, using weight machines or doing body-weight exercises. Space out your activities throughout the week. If you want to lose weight, or meet specific fitness goals, you may need to increase your physical activity time. One way to achieve all this is to go to a gym on say Mondays, Wednesdays and Fridays for one hour sessions of about 30 minutes of aerobic exercise and 30 minutes of strength training, do a ParkRun and or some high intensity work (on a stationary bike or powering bursts up hill) on Saturdays and go for walks or play golf or cut the lawn and do gardening on Sundays.

Recent research found that even a bit of regular physical activity goes a long way, spurts of exercise throughout the day are associated with significant reductions in disease risk. Researchers looked at the records of over 25,000 people with an average age of 62 who did not exercise regularly and followed them over the course of nearly seven years. Those who engaged in 2 or 3 minute bursts of reasonably intense exercise roughly three times a day, like speed-walking while commuting to work or rapidly climbing stairs, showed a nearly 50% reduction in cardiovascular mortality risk and about 40% reduction in the risk of dying from cancer as well as all causes of mortality, compared with those who did no vigorous bursts of exercise.

It seems that quick blasts of exercises that involve effort, performed repeatedly with short rest periods, can increase oxygen uptake and keep cardiac arteries from clogging, as well as power the heart to pump more blood and function better overall (especially when this is combined with eating the right foods).

Remember to check with your doctor before starting a new exercise program, especially if you haven't exercised for a long time, have chronic health problems, such as heart disease, diabetes or arthritis, or you have any concerns. All participants should give informed consent and may complete a Readiness Questionnaire. Par-Q

Drinking water is important to lubricate joints and tissues so they can be more elastic. Muscle cramps may result from dehydration.

Always follow a standard warm up procedure. Foam rollers may be used as part of a warm up or recovery program. Placing a foam roller under parts of your body and performing back and forth movements over the roller to exert pressure on soft tissues can help to improve flexibility.

Functional Movement

Movement patterns can have a major impact on our bodies. Genetically, the human body was designed to jump, run, swim, throw, and perform at a high level. However, through the demands of everyday life, stressors occur that produce negative impacts on our body's mechanics. As a result, pain, imbalances, asymmetries, and decreased function occur. By assessing basic movement patterns, we can attempt to head off problems and recover optimum function, mobility and stability.

To perform these tests you need an uncluttered doorway, some masking or electrical tape and a broom handle or long stick. Ideally ask someone to watch your 5 movement tests and give you helpful feedback.

Instructions: *this is an objective, 5 part test in which we look at a leg raises, bodyweight squat, a press up, shoulder and hip mobility. Each part is scored out of 2. Give yourself the full 2 points if you perform the movement almost perfectly, 1 point if it was not smooth or complete and 0 points if you could not do it or you felt pain.*

- Part 1 **Straight Leg Raise** – *Hip flexor stability and posterior chain mobility are shown together in this test.* Lie down on your back, in the doorway, with your hips between the door posts. Touch the door posts on either side and shuffle your body up or down until the middle fingers on both your hands are fully extended. Keeping your leg straight, lift the foot of one leg off the floor, point your toes and continue to raise your leg until it is at right angles to the floor (parallel to the door frame). Try not to bend your knee and do not allow the other leg to lift off the floor. Lower your leg slowly and try to do the same movement with the other leg.

- Part 2 **Seated rotation** – *to asses upper trunk stability* - sit cross legged close to, and facing, one of the door posts, with one foot on each side of the door post. Hold the broom stick horizontally across your collar bones, with both hands. With your back straight, rotate your upper body slowly left and then right and try to touch the post, on both sides, with the stick. Avoid the temptation to lean forward. Your spine should remain straight and upright.

- Part 3 **Overhead Squat Test** - *mobility, postural control, pelvic and core stability are well represented in a deep, overhead squat movement pattern.* Stand facing a closed door with your feet shoulder width apart and toes about 10cms from the door. Hold the broom stick high above your head (like a weightlifter). Keeping your knees and the stick away from the door, lower your bottom slowly to about ankle height (as far as you can comfortably) and then push back up to standing again. Award 2 points if your heels remain flat on the ground, your bottom is below your knees, and your arms are still almost vertical.

- Part 4 **Rotational Stabilization** - *to check core stability, muscle development, and body coordination.* Kneel on the floor, lean forward and place your palms on the floor below your shoulders, so that your back is roughly parallel to the floor. Stretch your left arm out in front of you until it is in a straight line with your back. Now do the same with your right leg – stretch it out behind you parallel to the floor. Stabilize, then try to touch your left elbow to your right knee, beneath your torso, and repeat this three times, then do the same with your right arm and left leg. Did you manage these movements without wobbling or over balancing? Did you stretch out fully then touch knees to elbows? If so give yourself 2 points, if you failed give yourself 0, 1 point if you did not stretch fully but did not wobble.

- Part 5 **Hurdle Step** – *to assess the bilateral mobility and stability of the hips, knees and ankles* - stick a tape horizontally across the doorway at a height equal to the top of your shins (ie below your knees). Standing with both feet together on one side of this hurdle and the broom stick resting horizontally on your shoulders, lift one foot up and over the tape progressively and place its heel on the floor on the other side before returning it. Do the same with the other foot. You should not touch the tape and the stick should remain horizontal and not touch the door posts. Note any differences or difficulties. 2 points for an almost perfect movement.

1) Functional Movement Tests

Movements	Points		
Straight leg raise	0	1	2
Seated rotation	0	1	2
Overhead squat	0	1	2
Rotational stability	0	1	2
Hurdle step	0	1	2
Totals			

Total score for all 5 functional movements = (/ 10)

2) Average Steps Per Day

If you have been wearing a smart watch (or carrying a smart phone or pedometer) recently you will be able to see how many steps per day you tend to do. You should note down the average number spread over the last few days.

Instructions: *award yourself points out of 10 based on the table below, for example if you do an average of 10,001 steps a day give yourself 8 points.*

Steps per Day	
Number of Steps	Points
Over 12,000	10
Over 11,000	9
Over 10,000	8
Over 9,000	7
Over 8,000	6
Over 7,000	5
Over 6,000	4
Over 5,000	3
Over 4,000	2
Over 3,000	1
Under 3,000	0

Score for Steps per day = (/10)

3) Sit and Reach Flexibility

This straightforward test is designed to measure the flexibility of your hamstrings and lower back. Flexibility refers to your ability to move joints and muscle fibres through their normal full ranges of motion, the more flexible you are, the better your range of motion and the less chance of stiffness and injury. If the fibres are short they limit the range of motion a joint will have. If they are at an optimal length and have enough elasticity, they allow the joint to move well.

Before you start, do some stretching and warming up.

Instructions: *Take your shoes off and sit on the floor with your back against a wall or door and your knees bent. Place a pen or pencil or other similar object in front of one of your heels so that as you straighten your legs and press the back of your knees down towards the floor, the object is pushed away from you. Your legs should be extended in front of you in a V shape, feet about 20 to 30 cms apart, toes pointing up, with the back of your knees (almost) touching the floor. Is this a comfortable position? Can you maintain it without too much pain? If yes, place your hands together, (one on top of the other), palms down, on the floor between your legs, and begin to stretch and reach forward slowly, without straining, towards (and past) your heels. Now sit back upright and place a second pen or pencil or similar object in front of your fingertips so that, as you stretch your hands forward along the floor, you push the object towards (and if possible past) your heels. At the point of your greatest reach, hold for a couple of seconds. See how far you have reached, in front of, or behind, the heel line. If you have trouble straightening your legs, you can ask a friend to help by holding your knees down flush with the floor as long as it is not too painful.*

Measurement: *Measure the distance between the two objects (the one at the heel line and the one your finger tips pushed). Take note of how far you reached relative to your heels. Use the table below to rate your score. For example, a man scores 6 points if he reaches 12 cms beyond his heels. A woman scores 5 points for that distance.*

Sit and Reach Flexibility Test		
Men (cms)	Women (cms)	Points
>30	>33	10
27 to 29	30 to 33	9
23 to 26	26 to 29	8
17 to 22	21 to 25	7
10 to 16	16 to 20	6
5 to 9	11 to 15	5
0 to 4	5 to 10	4
-4 to 0	4 to 0	3
-8 to -3	-7 to -1	2
-20 to -9	-14 to -8	1
< -21	<-15	0

Score for Sit and Reach Flexibility = (/10)

4) Balance on one leg

We have already noted that many of us are too sedentary these days, we work at a desk and spend most of the day sitting on chairs and couches. We used to spend far more time on our feet and it seems that our balance and health is suffering as a result. Standing is good for us and standing on one foot from time to time seems to double the benefits. Failures of balance and falls are the biggest causes of accidental deaths worldwide, after car crashes.

Balance requires a lot of coordination, it takes dynamic cues from your ears, eyes, nerves, joints and muscles. People with poor balance have been found to perform worse in tests of mental decline, suggesting a link with dementia.

Research studies show that people who find it difficult to balance on one leg are more likely to suffer from obesity, heart disease, high blood pressure, stroke, unhealthy blood fat profiles and are three times more likely to have Type 2 diabetes, yet balance assessment is not included in health checks usually.

Moreover, your ability to stand on one leg can be a powerful predictor of how long you will live. A 1999 study asked 2,760 men and women, in their 50s, to carry out 3 assessments: 1 grip strength, 2 how often they could stand upright from sitting in a minute, and 3 how long they could stand on one leg with their eyes closed. 13 years later these volunteers were invited to do the 3 tests again. While it turned out that all the tests provided some indication or prediction of how likely it was that a person would die from cancer or a heart attack, the researchers were surprised that the one-legged standing test came out on top. Those people who only managed to stand for two seconds or less on the earlier test were three times more likely to have died over the next 13 years than those who managed ten seconds or more.

Instructions: Stand with your feet about hip-width apart. Form a sort of T shape by lifting one foot off the ground and pointing it behind you (so that your whole leg is roughly parallel to the ground) while leaning forward and pointing your hands out in front of you. Hold this balance-on-one-leg position as long as you can. Then return to the starting position and repeat the movement on the other side.

Mark yourself out of 5 for each side (each leg).

Balance on one leg – Left Leg						
Time (seconds)	<10	11 - 30	31 - 50	51 - 100	101-200	>200
Points	0	1	2	3	4	5

Balance on one leg – Right Leg						
Time (seconds)	<10	11 - 30	31 - 50	51 - 100	101-200	>200
Points	0	1	2	3	4	5

Score for Balancing on one leg =   (out of 10)

Now try it with your eyes closed.

Standing on one leg with your eyes closed is far harder than with them open. A beginner does well if they can do it for 10 seconds, especially as they get older, but practice helps. You can teach your brain to do this exercise better. So, stand on one leg as often as you like and you may find your balance improves quickly. This will have beneficial effects on your confidence, your dancing, skating, skiing, surfing and the other sports you do. Is also good for your core strength.

5) The Wall Sit / Quadriceps Endurance

The quadriceps endurance or wall sit squat exercise works most of your lower body and major leg muscles. It builds muscular endurance, which delays fatigue and helps you to perform optimally for longer periods of time. It is sometimes known as the "devil's chair" because it seems so easy at first but, as time goes by, your thigh muscles take the strain and start to burn.

Even though the wall sit is an isometric or static exercise, it can still be considered a compound exercise as it requires numerous joints and muscles to work in unison. The main reason for doing this exercise (other than this test) is to increase your endurance. You will notice that you will be able to hold a wall sit for longer and longer periods the more you do it, especially if you practice one leg at a time. This exercise also increases your heart rate and burns quite a lot of calories.

Instructions: *Stand with your back to a wall and lean back so that your back is against the wall. Move your feet away from the wall and allow your back to slide down until you reach the point where your thighs are parallel to the floor. Make sure that your ankles are directly below your knees. Your thighs should be at right angles to your back and your shins.*

Measurement: *The test requires you to hold that position as long as you can, so start a timer as soon as you begin. (Stop if you feel nasty knee or back pain). Circle the number of seconds you lasted on the table below and award yourself the points out of 10 that you achieved.*

The Wall Sit or Quadriceps Endurance Test		
Men (seconds)	Women (seconds)	Points
> 170	> 140	10
130 to 169	110 to 139	9
100 to 129	90 to 109	8
90 to 99	80 to 89	7
80 to 89	70 to 79	6
70 to 79	60 to 69	5
60 to 69	50 to 59	4
50 to 59	40 to 49	3
40 to 49	30 to 39	2
31 to 39	21 to 29	1
< 30	< 20	0

Score for Wall Sit quad test = (/10)

6) Plank Test.

The Plank test (also known as the **Prone Bridge Test)**, is quite a simple fitness test of core muscle strength, which can also be used as a fitness exercise for improving core strength.

Instructions: Lie face down on the floor. Point your toes down and lift your body off the floor so that you are resting on your toes and elbows. Your elbows should be located below your shoulders. Your body should not be bent, in other words there should be a straight line from your heels to bottom to shoulders. Look down at the floor. You can clasp your hands together if you like. The aim of this test is to hold an elevated plank position for as long as possible.

Plank Test	
Time (in seconds)	Points
<10	0
10 to 20	1
21 to 30	2
31 to 50	3
51 to 70	4
71 to 99	5
100 to 140	6
141 to 180	7
181 to 240	8
241 to 300	9
>300	10

Score for Plank test = (/10)

7) Five Kilometre Walk / Jog / Run

There are several ways you can do this test: 1) join a local Parkrun, 2) use the GPS function on your smart watch, 3) walk or run round a 400 meter athletics running track 12 ½ times.

It is quite important to do some stretching and warm-up exercises before you start and it may be helpful to walk, jog or run with someone else so that they can pace you.

Instructions: Time yourself for this 5km distance and then check the table below to see how many points you gained in this test.

Five Kilometre walk / jog / run test										
Time (Mins)	>70	<70	<50	<45	<40	<35	<32	<29	<26	<23	<20
Points	0	1	2	3	4	5	6	7	8	9	10

Score for 5km walk / run = (/10)

8) QCT / Harvard Step Test

The Queen's college step test (QCT) and the Harvard Step Test are submaximal exercise tests that are used to measure cardio-respiratory fitness. The tests involve of 3 or 5 minutes of stepping up and down on a bench or step at a set rate of about 24 steps per minute. Advantages of this test include its simplicity, minimal cost, little need for advanced equipment and reasonably low risk for people who may have heart disease.

You will need: a step or bench about 40 cms (16 inches) high, a way to count pulse / heart beats such as a smart watch or oximeter or your fingertips, a metronome or app that gives you a way to time the frequency and regularity of the steps.

Instructions: *The Step Test is conducted as follows:*

- *Set your metronome at 96 beats per minute.*
- *Stand facing the bench or step,*
- *When ready, step up onto the bench and then down, one foot at a time, following the beat of the metronome.*
- *Maintain a steady four-beat cycle, and continue this pattern: up, up, down, down for 3 minutes.*
- *At the end of 3 minutes sit down and look at your smartwatch or oximeter to see what your pulse / heart rate is, (or if you do not have these devices, sit down and find your pulse on your wrist or neck with your finger tips and count it for 60 seconds). This is the* **"step test pulse rate".**
- *If you like you can take 3 more measurements – count the heart rate after 1 minute, 2 minutes and 3 minutes – to assess your recovery rate (ie how quickly your heart rate returns to normal – the fitter you get the quicker this will be).*

Step Test Pulse Rate		
Scores		Points
Men	Women	
Less than 82	Less than 90	10
82 to 91	90 to 98	9
92 to 98	99 to 107	8
99 to 107	108 to 116	7
108 to 116	117 to 123	6
117 to 125	124 to 132	5
126 to 134	133 to 141	4
135 to 143	142 to 150	3
144 to 152	151 to 159	2
153 to 162	160 to 168	1
Over 162	Over 168	0

Score for Step Test = (/10)

This test can also be used to estimate maximal oxygen consumption. The VO2 Max test was devised as a way to measure the Maximum (Max) amount or Volume (V) of Oxygen (O2) that a person can utilise during exercise. It is often used to gauge aerobic fitness and endurance. Our lungs absorb oxygen as we breathe, which is converted to energy to power our cells. The higher our VO2 Max, the more oxygen our body can consume to manage demanding aerobic activities and the lower our risk of death. The QCT and Harvard step test produce reasonably good estimations of maximum oxygen uptake, especially when a well-equipped laboratory is not available.

9) Standing Long Jump

The standing long jump is a two footed horizontal jump from a standing position. It tests explosive leg power.

Instructions: *after a warm up, place a broom stick on the floor (or stick a line of tape down). Holding a pen or pencil or similar object in one hand, stand behind the stick / line with your feet slightly apart. You are going to leap forward* *as far as you can, taking off on, and landing on, two feet. Bend your knees and then swing your arms forward as you jump to increase your forward propulsion. Jump as far forward as possible, landing on both feet without falling backwards. Place the pen or pencil behind your heels. You are allowed three attempts.*

Scoring: measure the distance from the take off line to the pen or pencil (the back of your heels on your best jump) and look up the table below to see how many points out of 10 your scored.

Standing Long Jump Test		
Men (Distance in cms)	Women (Distance in cms)	Points
<100	<100	0
100 to 140	111 to 120	1
141 to 170	121 to 130	2
171 to 190	131 to 140	3
191 to 200	141 to 150	4
201 to 210	151 to 160	5
211 to 220	161 to 170	6
221 to 230	171 to 180	7
231 to 240	181 to 190	8
241 to 250	191 to 200	9
>250	>200	10

Score for Standing Long Jump = (/10)

10) Push-up / Press-up test

Strength and endurance in the muscles of the upper body, specifically the chest, shoulders, triceps, and core are good indications of overall fitness and upper body strength. Power and stamina are important for many sports. A strong upper body is useful for performing everyday activities and movements, such as carrying luggage or picking up children, with ease and without risking injury. Another benefit that doing upper body exercises regularly can bring is that many people feel better if they are trim and muscular.

Push-ups or Press-ups are a good way to test and build upper body muscular strength and endurance. Push-ups are often used as a fitness assessment and to monitor progress during strength and fitness training, so this test can help you to track your upper body muscular endurance and fitness over time. The exercise engages muscles throughout the body, from head to toe, to maintain a constant rigid position

You lift nearly 75 percent of your total body weight with a standard push-up. Using a modified push-up position reduces this to about 60 percent of your total body weight.

If you have not already, perform a short warm up.

Instructions for the Standard Push-up Test which is the version of the test usually used for men.

- *Begin in a push-up position on hands and toes with hands shoulder-width apart and elbows fully extended.*
- *While keeping a straight line from the toes to hips, and to the shoulders, lower your body so your elbows bend to 90 degrees.*
- *Push back up to the start position.*
- *That is one rep.*
- *Continue with this form and complete as many reps as you can without breaking form.*
- *Note the total number of full push-ups completed.*

How to Score Your Results: *Having completed the test, compare your results to the numbers in the table below. These figures are derived from tried and tested standards including: "Essentials of Exercise Physiology," the YMCA's "The Y's Way to Physical Fitness," the National Strength and Conditioning Association's "NSCA's Essentials of Personal Training," and the American College of Sports Medicine's "ACSM's Guidelines for Exercise Testing and Prescription."*

Push-Up Fitness Test – Men					
Age: 20-29	Age: 30-39	Age: 40-49	Age: 50-59	Age: 60+	POINTS
55 or more	45 or more	40 or more	35 or more	30 or more	10
50-54	40-44	35-39	30-34	25-29	9
45-49	35-39	30-34	25-29	20-24	8
40-44	30-34	25-29	20-24	15-19	7
35-39	25-29	20-24	15-19	10-14	6
30-34	20-25	15-19	11-14	7-9	5
25-29	15-19	12-14	8-10	5-6	4
20-24	12-14	10-11	6 -7	4	3
15-19	10-11	8-9	5	3	2
14 or fewer	9 or fewer	7 or fewer	4 or fewer	2 or fewer	1
No attempt					0

Instructions for the Modified Push-up Test. *The modified version of the test is often used for women, because they tend to have less upper body strength than men. Instead of resting on hands and toes the modified version rests on hands and knees.*

- *Begin in a modified push-up position, on the hands and knees with hands shoulder-width apart and elbows fully extended.*
- *Create a straight line from the knees, to the hips, and to the shoulders.*
- *Lower your upper body so your elbows bend to 90 degrees, then push back up to the start position. Keep a straight line, do not bend up or down.*
- *That is one rep.*
- *Continue with this form and complete as many reps as you can without breaking form.*
- *Take note of the total number of modified push-ups completed.*

Push-Up Fitness Test - Women					
Age: 20-29	Age: 30-39	Age: 40-49	Age: 50-59	Age: 60+	POINTS
50 or more	40 or more	35 or more	30 or more	20 or more	10
44 - 49	37 - 40	30 - 34	26 - 29	17 -19	9
39 - 43	34 - 37	26 - 29	23 – 26	14 - 16	8
34 - 38	29 - 33	22 - 25	20 - 23	12, 13	7
28 - 33	24 - 28	18 - 21	16 - 19	10, 11	6
23 - 27	19 - 23	14 - 17	12 – 15	8, 9	5
17 - 22	14 - 18	10 - 13	9 – 11	6, 7	4
11 - 16	9 - 13	7 - 9	6 – 8	4, 5	3
6 – 10	5 - 8	4 - 6	3 - 5	2, 3	2
5 or fewer	4 or fewer	3 or fewer	2 or fewer	1 or fewer	1
No attempt					0

You can practise this exercise every day.

Score for Push-up test = (/10)

Total score for the Exercise section = (/100).

It is important to warm down after exercise and workouts. Massages can help to relax muscles by increasing blood flow, decreasing knots and keeping fascia (connective tissue that covers the body like a web), more pliable. Chapter 9 discusses exercise related issues in more detail.

Let's look at some useful terms and concepts.

Hypertrophy

Hypertrophy is a term for a physiological process that involves an increase in the size and/or volume of cells, tissues, or organs in response to a stimulus. In the context of exercise and fitness, hypertrophy is used to describe the growth of skeletal muscle tissue due to resistance training. Hypertrophy occurs when muscle fibres are subjected to mechanical stress and damage, which triggers a cascade of events that lead to the activation of cells which help repair and regenerate damaged muscle fibres. Over time, with consistent training and proper nutrition, these repaired muscle fibres become thicker and stronger, leading to hypertrophy.

There are several factors that can influence the degree of hypertrophy, including the intensity, volume, frequency, and type of exercise performed, as well as individual genetics, age, and gender. Generally, hypertrophy is maximized when exercises are performed with heavy weights and high volume, using a variety of exercises that target different muscle groups. Hypertrophy is a natural and necessary process for the growth and adaptation of skeletal muscle tissue in response to resistance. By understanding the underlying mechanisms and optimizing training variables, individuals can maximize their potential for hypertrophy and achieve desired fitness goals.

Atrophy

Atrophy is the opposite of hypertrophy, referring to the shrinkage or loss of cells, tissues, or organs in response to a decrease in their use, stimulation, or demand. It can occur in, and affect, various parts of the body, including muscles, bones, organs, and nerves, and can result from a range of factors, such as aging, disuse, malnutrition, injury, or disease. Muscular atrophy, also known as muscle wasting, is a common type of atrophy that occurs when there is a loss of muscle mass, strength, and function. It can be caused by several factors, such as prolonged bed rest, immobilization, reduced physical activity, nerve damage, and certain medical conditions, such as cancer, AIDS, and heart failure. Muscular atrophy can lead to a range of symptoms, including weakness, fatigue, loss of balance, and difficulty performing daily activities.

Another type of atrophy is brain atrophy, which is characterized by a decrease in the size and weight of the brain, as well as a loss of brain cells and connections. Brain atrophy can occur naturally as a result of aging or as a consequence of various neurological disorders, such as Alzheimer's disease, Parkinson's disease, multiple sclerosis, and stroke. Brain atrophy can cause a range of cognitive and behavioural symptoms, such as memory loss, confusion, mood changes, and difficulty with movement and coordination. Other types of atrophy include bone atrophy, which can lead to osteoporosis and increased risk of fractures, and organ atrophy, which can affect various organs, such as the heart, liver, and kidneys, and can cause a range of symptoms, depending on the affected organ.

Sarcopenia

Sarcopenia means "lack of flesh." It is the term for the progressive, loss of skeletal muscle mass and strength as we get older. Unfortunately, sarcopenia shortens life expectancy in those it affects. It can begin in our 30s or 40s and usually accelerates between the ages of 65 and 80. Rates vary, but we can lose 3% to 10% of our muscle mass every 10 years. Older people with vitamin D deficiency, insufficient calorie and protein intake, higher levels of inflammation and stress, and a sedentary lifestyle seem to be at most risk of sarcopenia. Studies show that sarcopenia can be slowed, and muscle loss decreased, with a healthy diet and regular exercise. The best treatment for sarcopenia is resistance and strength training. Using weights and resistance bands increases muscle strength and endurance. Nutrients such as omega 3, creatine, vitamins C, D and E, and glutamine may be beneficial in promoting healthy muscle mass. A decrease in the size and number of muscle fibres causes sarcopenia, whereas, with muscle atrophy there is a reduction in the size of the fibres, but the amount of fibres stays the same.

Autophagy

The word autophagy might be translated as "self-devouring", it is our body's way of cleaning out damaged cells to regenerate newer, healthier cells. It occurs when the body realises there isn't much food around, and starts rummaging through our cells, looking for anything we don't need. It clears out the junk, and recycles it into fuel, or new building materials, renewing our cells. Cells are the building blocks of every tissue and organ in your body and each cell contains parts that keep it functioning. Over time, these parts can become defective or stop working. Cancers start from defective cells that the body should recognize and remove. Autophagy is the process through which the body removes dysfunctional cells and recycles parts of them, so autophagy plays a role in preventing and treating cancer. Autophagy declines as we age, which means that cells that no longer work or may do harm are more likely to multiply. Some recent studies suggest that cancerous cells can be removed through autophagy. Intense exercise and fasting for 18 to 48 hours are ways to trigger autophagy. Foods that can help to induce autophagy include: green tea, coffee, ginger, onions, nuts, turmeric (curcumin), broccoli sprouts and some mushrooms.

Chapter 6

NUTRITION

What is the best diet?

The majority of life threatening and debilitating diseases are caused by our lifestyles and are avoidable. The biggest cause of early death in a growing number of countries is poor diet - it kills far more people than smoking or any other risk factor. The Global Burden of Disease Study cited diet as the number one cause of death and disability in the United States. The standard western diet results in dysbiosis, an imbalance where bad bacteria take over and increase our susceptibility to inflammatory diseases, colon cancer, metabolic syndrome, type 2 diabetes, and cardiovascular disease.

Autopsies and surgical operations on young people show that CVD starts at an early age. The arteries of most teenage accident, war, homicide, and suicide victims have fatty streaks that turn into plaques and become ticking time bombs that cause heart attacks and strokes. That is why we should not wait until our heart disease becomes symptomatic before we begin to treat it. We should reduce our LDL cholesterol through a diet that is low in saturated fat, eggs, meat, dairy, and junk.

So, in order to stop the epidemic of chronic diseases we have to change lifestyles, starting as early as possible. Can this be done? Well, in the 1960s, men living in Finland had the world's highest death rate from heart disease. Though tough, lean and rugged from jobs like farming and logging, they liked butter, whole milk, cheese, salt, sausage, and cigarettes. They only ate a fruit or vegetable occasionally. Anything green was dismissed as "food for animals." The North Karelia Project, promoted healthier behaviours by getting people to eat more fruits and vegetables and cutting saturated fat from their diet. Farmers diversify into crops such as berries. Bread companies lowered the salt and butter content of their recipes. A sausage maker, who had been defiant about keeping his pork fat ingredients, only switched to mushrooms after he had suffered a heart attack himself. Within 40 years the number of deaths from CVD had plunged by 82% and all-cause mortality by 45%. Finland has proved it is possible to reduce chronic disease and save lives. It shows us that if you can get everyone involved in a program that supports healthy choices: (growers and grocers, doctors and patients, schools and universities, service organizations and workplaces, government and sports clubs, influencers and the media), there can be rapid improvements.

The Good, the Bad and the Ugly

A plant-based diet can help to treat, prevent and in some cases reverse almost every one of the fifteen leading causes of death in developed countries. It can also allow us to be more active, slow down the aging process and, in essence, keep us younger for longer.

Obesity, diabetes and heart disease have become global health problems. The number of people diagnosed with diabetes has risen rapidly, affecting around 10% of the population in some parts of the world, and this dramatic increase have been attributed directly to poor dietary choices.

Research also shows that a well-balanced, plant-based diet can help our immune system, for example, doctors and nurses who were on a plant-based diet had a 70% lower rate of moderate to severe effects of the COVID virus than average, whereas those on a high meat, low carb diet had a 50% higher rate.

So what should we avoid, what foods constitute the most important sources of nutrients and in what proportions should we consume them?

While you can eat almost as much as you like of organic leafy, cruciferous and colourful vegetables, legumes and fruit, you need to restrict, (or eradicate), the amount of some items such as meats, fish, dairy products, sugar, salt, fizzy drinks, most man-made / artificial / refined foods and you need to cut out toxic and dangerous products like processed / smoked and burnt meat, trans-fats, most snacks, high sugar or fructose products, ultra-processed foods and those with long, complicated, lists of ingredients that contain preservatives and chemicals.

The World Health Organization has classified processed meats such as ham, bacon, salami and hot-dog frankfurters as Group 1 carcinogens (known to cause cancer) which means that there is strong evidence that processed meats cause cancer.

A 2021 systematic review and meta-analysis of meat consumption and risk of ischemic heart disease, that covered over 1.4 million cases, found that consuming just 50 grams a day (less than 2 ounces) of unprocessed red meat was associated with a 9% relative risk of heart disease and 50 grams of processed meat intake doubled that to an 18%. These risks rise with increased consumption. Low carb, low fruit, low veg, carnivore diets are unhealthy.

The human gut contains a remarkably diverse collection of microorganisms that help us to process what we eat, and the food we consume determines what kind of bacteria we grow in our gut. When we eat fibre-rich foods, the good, anti-inflammatory, fibre-munching organisms multiply. Good bacteria are nourished by vegetables, fruits, whole grains, and beans. Bad bacteria, those that contribute to disease, are fed by animal-based products, ultra-processed junk and fast food. Typical western diets can ruin our good gut flora and increase our risk of getting debilitating and killer diseases.

Recently published research confirms that the consumption of ultra-processed food is not only linked to cardiovascular disease, metabolic syndrome and obesity, but also with a 28% faster rate of global cognitive decline. Warning signs include products that have labels like "low calorie" and "low fat", with preservatives, chemicals, additives and substances you have not heard of.

It is a pity that only about 15% of the typical or standard diet in the USA is composed of reasonably healthy products, which probably helps to explain why so many Americans have chronic diseases. 19% is refined grains, 17% is added sugar, 23% is added fat, 26% is meat, dairy and eggs, 5% is vegetables, 4% is whole grains, 3% is fruit and 3% is beans and nuts. The USDA estimates that 63% of the Standard American Diet is composed of processed foods, 25% comes from animals and just 12% is from plants.

It turns out that the healthiest diet is also the most ethical and the most environmentally friendly.

It is estimated that one person who eats a diet that includes lots of animal products needs 2 acres of land to produce their food, but 2 acres can feed 12 people on a plant-based diet. The number of people on Earth has doubled in the last 50 years but the amount of meat we eat has tripled. About 150 million tonnes of seafood, 5 million horses, 28 million water buffalo, 325 million cows, 500 million goats, 600 million sheep, 630 million turkeys, 720 million geese, 1,400 million pigs, 3,300 million ducks, and 72,000 million chickens are killed every year to feed this growing appetite for flesh. It is estimated that 167,634 animals are slaughtered for consumption every second.

Research shows that modern farming methods cause damage to soil, habitats, fresh water supplies, oceans, and climates. Factory farming of animals produces environmental degradation including: deforestation, biodiversity loss, dead zones, erosion, genetic engineering, irrigation problems, pollutants, greenhouse gases, toxic chemical accumulation (eg Glyphosate), soil degradation, waste and the overuse of antibiotics leading to antimicrobial resistance.

The bulk of our diet should consist of legumes (beans, peas and lentils), leafy green and colourful vegetables (such as tomatoes, spinach, carrots, kale, cucumbers and beetroot), and should include fruit and berries, seeds, mushrooms, starchy vegetables (sweet potatoes, squash, parsnips), nuts and whole grains. Ideally we should eat a wide variety of fresh, plant-based food every day.

Flexitarian, whole-food, plant-based diet

While the ideal diet may include nothing but *unprocessed, unrefined, organic, fresh, locally produced, plant-based, wholefood*, many people find this is unsustainable. Research studies show that vegetarian diets are associated with reduced mortality but may not be embraced by everyone. Consuming a flexitarian diet that is dominated by plant-derived foods is usually more acceptable. A pro-vegetarian food pattern, emphasising preference for plant-derived nutrition but allowing for other foods, has been found to reduce the risks of obesity, all-cause illness and mortality. For many people decreasing their consumption of animal foods together with compensatory increases in plant-based foods is a relatively modest change which is realistic, affordable, and achievable. The flexitarian, pro-vegetarian diet does not require a radical shift to the exclusive consumption of plant foods. It is a gradual and often more acceptable approach which has been shown to translate to, and result in, better health and well-being for those who adopt it.

Microbiome

It is becoming clear that our microbiome is very important to our health. Microbes outnumber our human cells ten to one. We have over 100 trillion of them with thousands of different species. These include not only bacteria but fungi, parasites, and viruses.

Although microbes are so small that you need a microscope to see them, they contribute a great deal to our health and wellness. The largest numbers are found in our intestines. The microbiome has been called a supporting organ because it plays so many key roles in looking after the daily processes of our body. Our gut bacteria assist digestion, destroy harmful bacteria and help to control our immune system. Autoimmune diseases such as diabetes, rheumatoid arthritis, psoriasis, muscular dystrophy, multiple sclerosis, and fibromyalgia are associated with dysfunction in the microbiome.

To promote a healthy microbiome, eat lots of fibre, the more wide ranging and varied the better, ideally about 30 different types of plants a week. Vegetables and fruit are loaded with fibre which is consumed by the good bacteria in your gut. Cut out sugary processed foods. Monosaccharides are digested so quickly that we may starve our beneficial microbes. Hungry microbes may resort to munching the lining of our intestine. Probiotics are full of live bacteria that should populate our gut with good microbes. Try to avoid antibiotics because they do not recognise the difference between good and bad gut bacteria, antibiotics kill all bacteria. Avoid red meat. Instead eat organic or home grown: beans, lentils, whole grains, apples, pears, spinach, broccoli, garlic, leeks, onions, bananas, asparagus, kiwi fruit, berries, nuts, seeds, root vegetables and fermented foods.

Nutrition Assessment

The *More From Life* assessments of nutrition are in 10 parts. The first 6 of these include items we can eat as often as we like, the next 2 (numbers 7 and 8) we should be more careful with, limit our consumption of and be cautious about, and the last 2 (numbers 9 and 10) include items we should avoid, substances that, over time, are likely to be poisonous and bad for us.

The best way to keep track of what you consume is to keep a diary and record everything, including what and how much you eat. Using the following 10 tables, estimate the amount you have of each.

1) Green Leafy and Cruciferous Vegetables

Broccoli, kale, rocket/ arugula, Romaine lettuce, Swiss chard, collard greens, beet greens, water cress, microgreens, Bok choy, Brussels sprouts, cabbage, endive, cauliflower, turnip greens, radishes, wasabi. Ideally eat many of these raw in salads and smoothies, and choose organic.

Award yourself up to 10 points if you have been consuming the equivalent of about 3 cups of various cruciferous and leafy greens every day. 3 points for 1 cup and 6 points for 2 cups, the more variety the better.

Green Leafy and Cruciferous Vegetables											
Amount	None										Lots
Points	0	1	2	3	4	5	6	7	8	9	10

2) Other Vegetables

Sweet potatoes, tomatoes, bell peppers, carrots, asparagus, beetroot, onions, spring onions, parsnips, celery, potatoes, pumpkin, squashes, yams, cucumbers, courgettes, zucchini, aubergines, leeks, artichokes, purple potatoes, snap peas.

Award yourself up to 10 points if you have been eating 2 cups of these colour- ful vegetables per day. The more colours the better. Give yourself 5 points if you only typically eat about 1 cup a day.

Other Vegetables											
Amount	None										Lots
Points	0	1	2	3	4	5	6	7	8	9	10

3) Legumes

Split peas, lentils, kidney beans, broad beans, runner beans, pinto beans, navy beans, cannelloni beans, black beans, butter beans, French beans, borlotti beans, fava beans, lima beans, chick peas, hummus, edamame and soy beans. (Full of fibre, protein, and essential minerals).

Research confirms we should eat legumes every day – the long term benefits are excellent, in fact they may be the most important predictor of survival - if you want to increase your lifespan, eat beans. Judge your intake and award yourself points depending on the amount you normally consume. Give yourself up to 10 points if you eat 2 cups of legumes per day.

Legumes										
Amount	None									Lots
Points	0	1	2	3	4	5	6	7	8	9	10

4) Fruit and Berries

Apples, oranges, pears, bananas, melons, lemons, limes, guavas, cherries, peaches, tangerines, mangos, apricots, plums, olives, pomegranates, figs, kiwi fruits, rhubarb, persimmon, passion fruits, loquats, pineapple, avocados. Raspberries, blueberries, cherries, grapes, cranberries, blackcurrants, kumquats, amla and goji berries.

Eating fruit should be a both pleasure and a habit. Award yourself up to 10 points if you eat 3 handfuls of varieties of different fruit and about ½ a cup of berries each day. About 2 points for per item of fruit and 4 points for different berries.

Fruit and Berries										
Amount	None									Lots
Points	0	1	2	3	4	5	6	7	8	9	10

5) Whole Grains

Steel cut oats, whole oats, rolled oats, porridge, whole wheat, corn (maize), rye, bulgur (cracked wheat), millet, spelt, barley, buckwheat, quinoa, brown rice, popcorn, whole-grain and whole-wheat pasta and bread.

Award yourself up to 10 points if you have an average of about 3 cups of wholegrains each day. 3 points for 1 cup, 6 points for 2 cups.

Whole Grains											
Amount	None									Just right	
Points	0	1	2	3	4	5	6	7	8	9	10

6) Herbs, Spices, Mushrooms and Fermented

Garlic, turmeric, pepper, basil, oregano, ginger, chili, sage, thyme, rosemary, parsley, cumin, coriander / cilantro, curry powder, paprika, vanilla, horse radish, nutmeg, mustard, cardamom, cloves, dill, fenugreek, barberries, lemon-grass, peppermint, marjoram, allspice; Portobello, button, Shiitake, chanterelles, oyster, chestnut. pickles, kefir, kimchi, kombucha and sauerkraut.

Award yourself up to 10 points if you eat about a teaspoon of herbs and spices (especially if that includes garlic and turmeric) a day plus ½ of a cup of mushrooms (mushrooms add nutrients not found in other foods), plus occasional fermented foods, (the benefits of fermented foods are discussed in chapter 10), = about 3 points for each.

Herbs, spices, mushrooms and fermented											
Amount	None									Enough	
Points	0	1	2	3	4	5	6	7	8	9	10

7) Nuts and Seeds

Flax seeds, Chia seeds, pumpkin seeds, sunflower seeds, walnuts, Brazil nuts, cashews, pistachios, pine nuts, macadamia nuts, pecans, almonds, turmeric. A handful of nuts per day is plenty.

Award yourself up to 10 points if you usually (over the last few days) eat about 1 tablespoon of flax or chia seeds plus a ¼ cup of nuts per day, = up to 5 points for seeds and 5 points for nuts. (Flax seeds provide 10 times the lignans of other foods).

Nuts and Seeds										
Amount	None									Enough
Points	0	1	2	3	4	5	6	7	8	9	10

8) Treats

These are the foods that you should be cautious about, carefully control the amount you consume and eat occasionally such as: milk, cheese, fizzy drinks, "energy" bars, breakfast cereals, meat, (a portion of beef, chicken, pork, turkey), fish, shellfish, eggs, dates, fried potatoes, milk chocolate, biscuits, mayonnaise, salad cream.

You can have one of each of these treats every week. Subtract 1 point for every item you have after that from 10 points – (so if you had 2 energy bars, 2 portions of meat and 2 eggs subtract 3 points from 10 to give you 7 points).

Treats										
Amount	Too many									A few
Points	0	1	2	3	4	5	6	7	8	9	10

9) Products full of sugar, salt and refined grains.

Avoid these artificial, man-made, sweetened, processed and highly refined tempters: pastries, commercial cakes, croissants, donuts, microwave popcorn, artificial sweeteners, crisps, white bread, concentrated fruit juices, snacks and products that are full of sodium or high-fructose corn syrup, so called sports and energy drinks, candy bars, man-made products in packages, jars or boxes that contain preservatives.

Starting with 10 points, subtract 1 point for every item on this list that you have consumed during the last 7-days.

Products that are full of sugar, salt and refined grains											
Amount	Lots										V. Little
Points	0	1	2	3	4	5	6	7	8	9	10

10) Toxic and ultra-processed stuff

Includes poisons many of which the WHO ranks as carcinogenic, such as: spam, sausages, hot dogs, bacon, ham, salami, pates, corned beef, burgers, smoked / processed / burnt BBQ meat, deep fried foods, trans-fats, margarines, refined vegetable oil, palm oil, processed cheese, cream, ice cream, most pizzas, low-fat yogurts, fast foods.

Starting with 10 points, subtract 1 point for every item on this list that you have consumed during the last 7-days or so.

Toxic and ultra-processed foods											
Amount	Lots										V. Little
Points	0	1	2	3	4	5	6	7	8	9	10

Total score for the Nutrition section = (/100).

This set of assessments may sound complicated at first, but, for example, a lunch or dinner of:

- Vegetable soup and wholemeal or sourdough bread with hummus as a starter.
- Followed by a salad main course of rocket (arugula), carrots, spinach, split peas, spring onions, bell peppers, tomatoes and sliced apple with a sprinkle of walnuts, pumpkin seeds, flax seeds and goji berries and a topping of some balsamic vinegar and maybe mustard.
- Then some fruit for dessert.

This covers many of your daily needs in one meal.

A simpler way to put this is to say that about half the plate should contain vegetables, a quarter should be whole grains and a quarter legumes / beans; with fruit on the side.

You are what you eat - Food can be medicine

Eat **organic, whole, unprocessed, plant-based food** as much as possible. Avoid animal products (beef, pork, lamb, chicken, turkey, fish, milk, eggs, ...). Keep an eye on your intake of salt, sugar and preservatives (read the packets). Minimise your exposure to pollutants and contaminants such as weed killers (glyphosate), agro-chemicals, pesticides, dioxins, mercury, heavy metals and GM (Genetically Modified) products.

Fibre, also known as "roughage", is vital to our health yet most of us do not get enough fibre in our diets. It helps to keep our gut microbiome digestive system working well. Research shows that the bacteria and other micro-organisms in our gut are very important for our physical and mental well-being. Eating plenty of fibre is associated with a lower risk of heart disease, stroke, type 2 diabetes and bowel cancer. Choosing foods with fibre also helps to make us feel fuller, keeps us regular and prevents constipation. Government guidelines say our dietary fibre intake should be 30 grams (ideally 50g) a day. There is no fibre in meat or dairy or eggs or sugar. Beans are a good source.

Fibre is found in all types of plant-based foods, including: fruit, vegetables, pulses and grains.

- Legumes: Navy beans, Split peas, Pinto beans, Kidney beans, Chickpeas, Soybeans, Lentils.

- Vegetables: Broccoli Flowerets, Brussels sprouts, Garlic, Asparagus, Tomato, Onions, Artichokes, Squash, Green peas, Turnip greens, Carrots, Cauliflower, Sweet potato.

- Fruit: Avocados, Apples, strawberries, Bananas, Raspberries.

- Nuts & Seeds: Almonds, Pecans, Peanuts, Walnuts, Chia seeds.

- Whole Grains: Barley, Whole grain pasta and rice, Quinoa, Oats, Popcorn.

The **glycaemic index** (GI) is a numerical measure of how quickly and how much a particular food raises blood sugar levels. Foods with a higher GI are those that are full of refined carbohydrates and sugars, such as white bread, pasta, and sugary drinks whereas foods with a lower GI are those that are high in fibre, such as whole grains, vegetables, and legumes. People with diabetes can reduce spikes in their blood sugar levels and the risk of complications by choosing foods with a lower GI. However, GI is just one factor to consider when choosing foods, other factors, such as nutrient content of a food, volume of protein and fat, amount of food consumed, timing of meals, and individual differences in insulin sensitivity, should also be taken into account.

So it is important to be careful with **refined carbohydrates**, cut down or eliminate the consumption of products containing sugars, concentrated sweeteners, white flour and white rice, especially as these can be addictive.

Many myths surround protein. Firstly, it is completely untrue that you must get protein from animals (meat, eggs, dairy and fish). Second it is highly unlikely that we might be protein deficient. Beans / legumes, such as soy, edamame and tofu, broccoli, nuts, seeds and oats provide plenty of protein. Aim to consume about 1 gram of protein for every kg you weigh (some suggest 1.2 grams).

The more processing a food gets the less healthy it becomes.

Maximise your intake of anti-oxidants and phytochemicals. Choose the rainbow of colours and eat a wide variety of fruit, vegetables and beans.

Eat plenty of rocket (arugula), beetroot, broccoli, spinach, kale, carrots and garlic to boost your Nitric Oxide levels and look after your blood vessels, muscles and immune system.

Eliminate trans fats and cut down on fried foods.

More healthy fats include: avocados, walnuts and seeds which also contribute omega 3.

Do not overeat. Try not to eat so much that you feel full or bloated.

For any meal you prepare, ask yourself – How can I make this healthier?

Dr. Michael Greger's, NutritionFacts.org, Daily Dozen app is a free and very useful tool to help you keep track of your nutrition.

Alongside these recommendations it is well known that we should keep ourselves properly hydrated, control our alcohol intake to about 1 drink a day and not smoke, (these are discussed in chapter 7).

Chapter 7

Habits ("The Fifth Quarter")

So far, we have covered a wide range of health and well-being factors but four significantly important assessments have not been dealt with. These are: smoking (air quality), alcohol consumption, hydration and sleep. They are included in this chapter.

1) Smoking, Vaping and Air pollution

We noted in Chapter 2 that smoking is the one lifestyle habit that affects peoples' health more than any other. Research studies confirm that smoking is one of the most significant potential killers that we have control over. It causes a remarkable variety of horrible adverse effects on the body, including inflammation and decreased immune function. Smoking is linked to many nasty conditions and diseases (including diabetes, arthritis, cancer, heart attacks and strokes), harms most of the body's organs and is the leading cause of preventable death in many countries. It increases your risk of developing more than 50 serious health conditions, causes about 90% of all lung cancer deaths and about 80% of all deaths from chronic obstructive pulmonary disease (COPD).

In fact, smoking can cause cancer almost anywhere in your body, including: bladder, blood (acute myeloid leukaemia), cervix, colon and rectum (colorectal), oesophagus, kidney and ureter, larynx, liver, oropharynx (includes parts of the throat, tongue, soft palate, and the tonsils), pancreas, stomach, trachea, bronchus, and lung. If nobody smoked, one of every three cancer deaths would not happen.

Smoking is often responsible for other problems: such as making it harder for a woman to become pregnant and affecting a baby's health. It increases the chance of ectopic pregnancy, early delivery, stillbirth, low birth weight, sudden infant death syndrome and cot death. Smoking can also cause erectile dysfunction, reduce men's sperm fertility and increase risks for birth defects and miscarriage.

The risk of developing type 2 diabetes is 30% to 40% higher for smokers than non-smokers.

Smoking affects the health of your teeth and gums and increases your risk for cataracts. It can also cause age-related macular degeneration (AMD) and rheumatoid arthritis. Women who smoke tend to develop weaker bones and are at greater risk of fractures.

Quitting smoking lowers your risk for these diseases dramatically and can add years to your life.

Instructions: *Award yourself 50 points if you do not smoke. Subtract 10 points for every smoke you have in a week, (ie if you smoke 3 cigarettes or cigars in one week subtract 30 from the 50 points = 20). Subtract 10 points if you are in an environment in which you receive second hand smoke or high levels of air pollution, (20 points if both of these apply).*

Smoking and Air Pollution						
Items Smoked / Pollution	>5	4	3	2	1	0
Points	0	10	20	30	40	50

Score for Smoking assessment = (/50)

2) Alcohol and Drugs

Alcohol has been produced and consumed by humans for almost 10,000 years, but drinking too much alcohol harms our health. It shortens people's lives. It can be addictive and cause people to act in ways they regret. Excessive drinking is responsible for about 1 in 5 deaths among adults aged 20-49 years.

Over time, excessive alcohol use can lead to weakening of the immune system, the development of chronic diseases and other serious problems. The long-term health risks of drinking too much include: developing high blood pressure, gout, heart disease, stroke, dementia, liver disease and digestive problems. Breast, throat, mouth, oesophagus, voice box, liver, colon, and rectal cancers. Mental health issues, including depression and anxiety, learning and memory problems. Social and job-related problems and alcohol dependence.

Count your alcohol units. Current recommendations suggest we should drink no more than 14 units per week. So you should aim to average no more than one glass of beer (330ml), or wine (125ml) or spirits (50ml) per day. (A bottle of wine has about 10 units, a can of beer has about 2.5 units and a bottle of spirits has about 30 units).

Like alcohol, drug use can lead to dependence and addiction, injury and accidents, health problems, sleep issues, and more. Long term health impacts such as liver, kidney and heart problems or cancer (depending on the type of drug used and how frequently it is used), dental health problems (cavities and gum disease), mental health issues such as anxiety and depression. Drug use affects you and those close to you. Social consequences include: dropping out of school, job loss, hospitalisation, legal problems and arrests, troubled relationships, and being the perpetrator or victim of abuse.

Instructions: *For alcohol, start with 30 points then Subtract 4 points for every 1 unit over 14 units per week. In other words if you drink about 20 units per week (2 bottles of wine) you should subtract 24 points giving you an alcohol score of 6.*

For drug use rate yourself by consideration of the factors and consequences mentioned above.

Alcohol Consumption (in Units per Week)								
Units	>21	21	20	19	18	17	16	15	14
Points	0	2	6	10	14	18	22	26	30

Score for Alcohol consumption = (/30)

3) Hydration

Drinking enough water every day is essential. We are told to consume about 2 to 4 litres of fluids a day. Some of this fluid will come from the food we eat, especially if we consume a lot of fruit and vegetables – which contain a lot of water. Traditionally (since 1921, so for the last 100 years or so) we have been advised to drink about 8 glasses of water a day (based on rather flimsy evidence). One glass is equal to 250ml or about 8 fluid ounces (US). Clearly this recommendation is not a universal requirement – we all need different amounts. Nutritionists suggest we should aim to drink at least 1 litre of water per day. The rest can be water with fruit or soups or herbal teas.

Not drinking enough water has been associated, (especially in those people who have unhealthy lifestyles such as poor diets and little exercise), with heat stroke, heart disease, lung disorders, kidney disease, kidney stones, bladder and colon cancer, urinary tract infections, constipation, decreased immune function, cataract formation and fractures.

The factors that influence our bodies hydration levels, include:

- our age, older people are more vulnerable to dehydration so it is important to make sure they are drinking regularly,
- our size, the larger we are the more fluid we need,
- our diet, vegetarians tend to require less water as they get a lot of their fluids from the food they consume,
- the climate, we need more water in hot weather,
- our consumption of alcohol, consuming stronger types of alcohol dehydrates us, so when we drink wine and spirits, we should remember to consume more water. Beer does not seem to have the same dehydration effect.
- the amount we exercise. We can lose a lot of water when we sweat, so it is important to replace it and certain electrolytes during and after exercise,
- air conditioners suck moisture out of a room to bring down the humidity,
- dehydration may occur when we are ill, especially if we have fever, vomiting or diarrhoea.

If you are not sure how to determine how hydrated you are a good ready reckoner is to look at your urine: the more light coloured = the better hydrated, the darker and deeper coloured = the more dehydrated you are. Dark, strong-smelling urine is a sign of dehydration and can be used as an indicator that we need to drink more. Other signs of dehydration can include: feeling thirsty, fatigue, brain fog, dry mouth, inelastic skin, cracked lips, muscle cramps, palpitations, fainting, headaches, light headedness and dizziness.

Drink water flavoured with berries, apple cider vinegar, orange, lemon or lime juice or sparkling water, but avoid sugar sweetened drinks. Start the day by squeezing the juice from a lemon and adding it to a glass of water. Create fresh soups and broths. Make a habit of drinking water with your meals. Carry a reusable water container with you so that it is always handy and you become used to topping up throughout the day.

Can you drink too much water? Our kidneys can eliminate up to 1 litre of fluid per hour so drinking a lot more than that could cause hyponatremia in some people. There are very rare cases of fatal water intoxication where a person has drunk seven litres in three hours or less.

It is important (at least for the first few days until you get the hang of it) that you keep a careful note of everything you drink each day, the amount, the time of day and whether it is water, fizzy drinks, coffee, tea or alcohol. It may surprise you. Record the amount of each that you drink typically. Add them all up to see how much you drink per day. You should drink more water than anything else.

Instructions: *Give yourself a score out of 10 for how well you stay hydrated. For example, if you keep yourself well hydrated, your pee is always very pale coloured and you drink at least 1 litre of water a day if you are a woman, or about 1.5 litres of water a day if you are a man, award yourself the maximum 10 points (see columns 1 and 2 in the table below). Add about 0.5 to 1 litre to these amounts if you live in a hot climate and / or exercise a lot and / or do not eat a lot of fruit and vegetables (columns 3 and 4). Add a bit more if you drink wine and spirits and / or have diarrhoea or sickness.*

Hydration (water intake measured in litres)				
1	2	3	4	
Cooler weather, little exercise, vegetarian diet		Hotter weather, more exercise, less fruit & vegetables		Points
Men	Women	Men	Women	
>2.0	>1.5	>3	>2	10
>1.9	>1.3	> 2.7	>1.8	9
>1.7	>1.2	> 2.4	>1.6	8
>1.5	>1.1	> 2.1	>1.4	7
>1.3	>0.9	> 1.8	>1.2	6
>1.1	>0.8	> 1.5	>1.0	5
>0.9	>0.7	> 1.2	>0.8	4
>0.7	>0.5	> 0.9	>0.6	3
>0.5	>0.3	> 0.6	>0.4	2
>0.3	>0.2	> 0.3	>0.2	1
<0.3	<0.2	< 0.3	<0.2	0

Adjust your fluid intake. If necessary, reduce alcohol intake and bring other fluids (especially water) up to the recommended 2 to 3 litres per day.

Score for Hydration = (/10)

4) Sleep

Sleep is vital, we need to rest every day to stay healthy. During sleep, many of the body's tissues and organs are recovering, repairing, rebuilding and restoring the immune, nervous, skeletal, and muscular systems. These are functions and processes that maintain mood, memory, and cognitive function, and play an important role in the endocrine and immune systems. Even small reductions in the sleep we need can cause fatigue, lack of energy, slowed thinking, reduced attention span, lower sex drive, poor balance, accidents, bad decision making, stress, anxiety, and irritability. Sleep deprivation can also cause depression, obesity and cardio vascular problems and is used by torturers.

Research shows that those who only get 4 or 5 hours sleep per night tend to have raised: blood pressure, resting heart rate, blood sugar level and have a greater risk of Alzheimer's disease. Alcohol is a sedative which blocks REM sleep. Sleep timing depends greatly on hormonal signals from a complex neuro-chemical system, named the circadian clock, which uses signals from the environment to create an internal rhythm. The circadian clock exerts constant influence on our body and affects the ideal timing of restorative sleep episodes. Sleepiness increases during the night but modern life may disconnect or de-synchronise us from our internal circadian clock, due for example to night shift working, long-distance travel, and the effects of indoor lighting.

Those people who get enough sleep have stronger immune systems and turn out to be about three times more likely to beat infections. To reduce the risk of cancer, stroke, and heart disease we need just the right amount – not too much or too little. Research studies indicate that, to maximise well-being and longevity, the ideal amount for many people is about 7 to 8 hours per night.

Instructions: *Select a number from 0 to 10 for your assessment of the duration and quality of sleep you have experienced during the past 7-days or so, in other words award more points if you usually have a good night's sleep that makes you feel properly rested.*

Sleep	
Quality and Duration of your sleep	Points
Fabulous sleep, really rested and relaxed	10
Good but not quite fully rested, woke a bit early	9
OK but less than 7 hours of sleep, a bit restless	8
Too much – over 10 hours sleep	7
Not enough sleep, feeling tired a lot of the time	6
Tossing and turning all night, nightmares	5
About 4 hours of sleep, really need to catch up	4
Broken sleep pattern, just about 3 hours sleep	3
About 1 or 2 hours of sleep, very distracted	2
Sleep deprived for many days	1
No sleep, cannot sleep, stressed and agitated	0

Score for Sleep assessment = (/10)

Total score for the Habits section = (/ 100)

Your More From Life total score = (/500).

Chapter 8

Putting It All Together

When you have tried the tests and assessments in the previous 5 chapters (Mind, Body, Exercise, Nutrition and Central issues) and become more aware of, and knowledgeable about, these different aspects of your current health and well-being, you can reflect on your results and answers and the extensive amount of data that has been generated, to gain insights, learn about yourself and consider what all this means for you.

Your More From Life Score

Adding the scores from the 5 chapters together gives you your first *More From Life* total score. (Each section is worth 100 points so the total is out of 500). Now you can look back on the results overall.

- What parts and assessments did you score well in and which parts and tests gave you your lowest points?
- Was this what you expected? Were there surprises?
- Which scores could you improve and what parts do you need to work on?
- Which evaluations or indicators should you do something about?
- Are you keen to have another go at some of the Exercise / Fitness tests or the Body, medical health assessments or the

Mind mental health section or the Nutrition / diet part, or all of them!

It is time to take the **One Week Challenge**. The idea is to adopt a set of recommendations for a week and see what effects they have. People who have taken this **One Week Challenge** previously have reported improvements to their overall score of around 10% on average. Several of them made important changes to their lifestyle, as a result, and halted or reversed worrying trends.

Follow these guidelines and try to stick to, and carry out, all the suggestions on the list below.

The One Week Challenge

1. Move more and keep active as much as possible. Walk don't drive, climb stairs instead of taking the lift / elevator. Make sure you achieve an **average of 10,000 steps per day**.

2. Try to do **20 to 40 minutes of strength training and reasonably vigorous exercise,** that uses your muscles and raises your heart rate, every day. Warm-up by stretching and dancing or jogging on the spot, then exercise for a half hour. You can go ahead and do more than this, or push yourself a bit harder, if you like.

3. Try meditation, mindfulness or Yoga or get some peaceful, quiet time for at least **10 minutes every day**. Aim to get 8 hours sleep.

4. Follow a **balanced, whole food, plant-based diet**. For one week do not eat any processed meat (bacon, ham, sausages, peperoni) or fast food, or ice cream or cakes or ultra-processed foods. Avoid animal products as much as possible and just eat cooked and raw vegetables, whole grains, beans, seeds, nuts and fruit.

5. Do **NOT smoke or drink alcohol** for the duration of the challenge. Drink plenty of water.

6. **Be a good example.** Do something nice and / or make a special effort to help someone else every day. Be kind. Do things they and you feel good about, things to be proud of. Aim to be altruistic, empathetic, compassionate and helpful. Listen, communicate and offer support. Have a sense of purpose.

7. **Nurture relationships.** Spend time with friends and family. Give and receive love. Join up and connect with others. Become part of, and enhance, communities.

8. **Joy and enjoy.** Try to see the good, positive, optimistic and joyful in everything. Appreciate life. There is an old saying that goes – "*Two men looked through prison bars, one saw mud the other saw stars*".

Notes and Guidelines

1) Steps and Zone Two

Easy ways to track how many steps you do per day include: wearing a smart watch or keeping your phone with you wherever you go or carrying a pedometer. If you like, you may do what is called Zone 2 training, which means exercising just above the easy zone, for example faster walking than ordinary walking pace to develop aerobic fitness, burn some fat and lower resting heart rate. Inexpensive and effective ways to get good exercise include climbing and descending flights of stairs and loading a rucksack or wheelbarrow with about 10kgs and going for a walk. A good indicator of how hard you are working is your breathing: you should be able to have a conversation, but singing and whistling will be difficult.

2) Active Strength Exercise

Do some strength training at least 2 or 3 times a week along with vigorous exercise on the other days such as: jogging, dancing, skipping, running, cycling, (including treadmills, stationary bikes and ellipticals), swimming, playing football, squash, tennis, table tennis, badminton, horse riding, kayaking, skiing, swimming, ice skating, digging the garden, squats, push ups, burpees, farmer carries, resistance training, gym workouts, aerobic classes, chopping wood, vigorous housework! Make your muscles work!

It has been suggested that there are 4 different aspects to consider about exercise. These are summarised by the acronym **TIFT = Type** (the type of exercise you choose), **Intensity** (the intensity of your exercise), **Frequency** (how often you exercise), and **Time** (how long you exercise). You may like to talk to a trainer about strength training and the most appropriate way forward. Practice some of the tests in chapter 5 such as functional movements, press ups, wall sit, one leg balance, sit & reach flexibility and the plank. Take it easy to start with, (especially if you have not been doing very much exercise recently) and build up to a level you are comfortable with. Slow down if you become breathless and stop if you sense pain or feel dizzy.

- Phase 1 = Stay active, walk and do some low-level activity every waking hour. Aim to get at least 30 minutes essential exercise that raises your pulse rate a bit, every day.

- Phase 2 = More effort, jog or cycle or swim at a faster rate that demands more effort and makes you breathe more deeply and increases your heart rate by 50% to 70% above resting.

- Phase 3 = Play football or badminton or basketball or hockey or mountain biking or judo or another sport that makes demands of you.

- Phase 4 = If you want to push yourself even harder try HIIT training, 3 or 4 short bursts of high intensity effort with the same amount of rest in between. Use battle ropes or stair-climber or a stationary bike to work as hard as you can for 30 seconds to 3 minutes. Alternatively run with a backpack, cycle fast uphill, or swim with a weight belt. Remember to warm up and cool down properly.

3) Meditation

Research suggests that meditation and mindfulness can be good for us, it helps us have a healthier relationship with ourselves and with others. Over 8,000 studies have been conducted that seem to show that meditation and mindfulness can improve sleep, learning and memory, reduce pain, anxiety and stress, help our autoimmune system and enhance our mood.

It does not work for everyone but taking a few peaceful, relaxing and calm minutes out of our busy day is unlikely to be harmful.

In mindfulness meditation, we can pay attention to our breathing and the breaths we take, as they go in and out, we notice when our mind wanders and learn how to return our mind to the breathing. When we pay attention to our breathing we can stay more in the present moment, we, as it were, anchor ourselves in the here and now, on purpose, without judgement.

To begin a mindfulness meditation, find a place to sit that feels calm and quiet, somewhere where you can relax. Set a time limit of say 10 minutes. Sit with your feet on the floor and your arms resting comfortably. Notice and feel your breathing, follow the sensation of your breaths as they go in and out. Your mind will inevitably wander and your attention will divert away from your breathing. Be kind to your wandering mind and return your thoughts to your breathing. Do not judge yourself badly or worry about the thoughts that crept in and intervened. Simply redirect and return your attention to your breath.

Take a deep inhale, expanding your tummy, then exhale slowly, elongating the out-breath as your belly contracts. Where do you feel your breath most? In your abdomen? In your nose? Try to keep your attention on inhaling and exhaling. When your mind wanders, bring it back, with kindness and patience.

Continue to practice bringing your attention to your breath, and back to the breath when you notice your attention has wandered. When you are ready, open your eyes and lift your gaze gently. Notice your present thoughts and emotions, how your body feels and any sounds around you.

When we experience distractions during meditation we realise how much time we, as it were, live in our heads, on automatic pilot, letting our thoughts go hither and thither, thinking about issues and problems, going over old ground again and again, wondering if we forgot to do something or worrying, looking back to the past or imagining the future, almost out of control, and not being present in the moment.

One of the reasons we should practice and learn meditation and mindfulness is to recognise when our minds are occupied (and sometimes overwhelmed) by their normal everyday acrobatics and choose to take a pause from that for a little while so we can focus on what we would like to think about. The process does not wipe our mind clear of all the countless, endless thoughts that erupt constantly in our brains, it helps us to be calmer and to focus and to control needless worries.

4) Follow a well-balanced, whole food, plant-based diet.

We have already noted that eating a well-balanced diet is essential to keep us at our best. Research shows that many ailments and diseases are due to poor diet. It is acknowledged that most heart disease, hypertension, strokes, diabetes type 2, certain types of cancer, arthritis, and possibly Alzheimer's are caused by a bad diet and that changing to a better diet can treat, prevent and in some cases reverse these diseases.

Base your choices of what to eat on the suggestions in Chapter 6. Consume a balance of legumes, fruit and vegetables, especially fresh, organic, plant-based wholefoods. Monitor and control your consumption of processed foods and animal products (avoid them as much as possible) and **cut out** the poisonous, carcinogenic and unhealthy stuff (such as fast food, bacon, sausages, salami, ham, hot dogs, margarine, white bread, croissants, pastries, cakes, donuts, cheesy meaty pizzas and deep-fried snacks).

Base your diet on the following:

- **Legumes** are excellent sources of protein, fibre, potassium, folate, iron and zinc. They are inexpensive, easy to prepare and among the most healthy and nutritious foods you can eat. Legumes include beans (such as: kidney, black, broad, runner, cannelloni, butter, soy, pinto, lima and soy), peas, lentils and chickpeas. Fortified soy milk is a reliable source of vitamins D and B12. There is a range of soy products such as tofu, tempeh and veggie burgers. Aim for at least 2 handfuls per day.

- **Fruits** have no cholesterol and most are low in calories, fat and sodium. They provide many essential nutrients including fibre, vitamin C, folate antioxidants and potassium. Fruit fibre and phytonutrients inhibit the transportation of sugars through the intestinal wall into our blood stream, slows the release of sugar and blunts potential fructose glycaemic spikes. They can be fresh, canned (avoid the syrup), or frozen. Aim to have at least 3 handfuls per day.

- **Berries** in all their colourful, delicious glory are protective little powerhouses. They are the most health giving of fruits, second only to herbs and spices as the most anti-oxidant packed food, (over fifty times more anti-oxidants than animal-based foods). Blueberries improve cognitive performance, (the more the better) and delay the aging of the brain by as much as 2 ½ years. Blueberries also feed our good bacteria, they are a natural probiotic. They help to reduce artery stiffness and boost the natural killer cells that defend us against infections and cancer. Put some in your breakfast or smoothie or pudding every day or eat them on their own as a snack – nature's sweets.

- **Vegetables** are also low in fat and calories and have no cholesterol. They are important sources of protein and are full of many nutrients including: potassium, fibre, folate, vitamin A and vitamin C. Green leafy vegetables like: rocket (arugula), broccoli, bok choy, collard greens, mustard greens, turnip greens and kale provide essential nutrients such as calcium, iron and nitrites. Aim to have 4 or more handfuls a day. They can be raw, juiced, pureed and or cooked. Beetroot, carrots and sweet potatoes are also wonderful foods. Consume a wide variety of types and colours to obtain the best range of carotenoids, flavonoids and other phytochemicals.

- **Whole grains** are important for fibre, B vitamins, thiamine, riboflavin, niacin, folate, iron, potassium, magnesium and selenium. Brown rice, quinoa, corn, millet, buckwheat, bulgur and oatmeal and all good whole grain choices. Fibre fills you up, removing it makes it far easier to eat too much junk. When whole wheat is processed into white flour, or brown rice into white rice, the fibre and bran are removed, turning "good carbs" into "bad carbs". Bad carbs are absorbed quickly causing your blood sugar to rise rapidly and making your pancreas secrete insulin to bring it back down – maybe too far. As a result, you may feel lethargic and crave more bad carbs = a vicious circle. Secreting too much insulin might lead to insulin resistance and diabetes, it also accelerates the conversion of calories into triglycerides, which is how your body stores fat. So you may consume a lot of calories that do not fill you up but add extra weight and fat. Aim to have about 3 to 5 handfuls of whole grains a day.

- **Nuts and seeds** are amazing foods that can add years to your life. The Global Burden of Disease Study calculated that not eating enough nuts and seeds was the third leading risk factor for disability and death in the world. Nuts and seeds are thought to reduce the risk of dying from heart disease, stroke, cancer, respiratory diseases, diabetes and infections. Nuts can help lower cholesterol and oxidation, as well as improve our arterial function and blood sugar levels. Just a few small servings of nuts a week may increase our lifespan and lower our cancer risk. They are a good source of fibre, omega 3 fats and plant protein and are a nutritious, quick and convenient snack. Walnuts, pistachios, almonds, hazelnuts, Brazil nuts, macadamia, pecans, cashews, and pumpkin, flax, sesame, hemp, sunflower and chia seeds. Aim to have an ounce or small handful a day.

Sample Menu Suggestions	
Breakfast	Oatmeal or sugar free Muesli with cranberries/ blueberries / raspberries Porridge with maple syrup and ground flaxseed Melon with wholewheat toast and hummus or peanut butter
Lunch	Green Juice or Smoothie* Homemade soup with sourdough bread Bean Salad
Dinner	Roast vegetables or Stews or Curry or Chili or Stir fry or Casseroles or "Bolognese" type tomato-based meal with: Beans, peas and lentils, broccoli, onions, spinach, peppers, sweet potato, carrot, mushrooms, parsnips, Brussel sprouts, cauliflower, beetroot, leeks, kale, butternut squash, pumpkin, courgette, green beans, sweet corn, scallions, tomatoes, cabbage, Tofu, sauerkraut. With brown rice, wholemeal pasta, couscous, quinoa, millet, roasted sweet potatoes.
Flavour and extras	Garlic, pepper, Himalayan salt, turmeric, ginger, sage, basil, oregano, thyme, mint, fenugreek, herbs de Provence, paprika, chili, pesto, tamari, balsamic vinegar, apple cider vinegar, lemon juice, red or white wine, nutritional yeast, soy sauce, crushed walnuts, almond flakes, pumpkin seeds, pine nuts, maple syrup, coconut milk, olive oil, mustard, curry powder, cumin, coriander, mixed spices.
Snacks	Nuts, seeds, olives, celery, carrots, avocado, apples, oranges, tangerines, grapes, bananas, mangos, kiwi fruit, pears, plums, apricots, peaches, pineapple, figs, cherries. Dark chocolate
Liquids	Water, teas (green, black, rooibos, hibiscus), coffee, non-dairy milks

Juicing and Smoothies

Slow juicing, or blending a smoothie of, fruit and vegetables, that would otherwise take a long time to eat, may help our bodies to gain essential vitamins, minerals and antioxidants that it can digest easily. Antioxidants help to repair and prevent the cell damage caused by free radicals that are linked to cancer and heart-related illnesses. Smoothies can increase fibre intake, contribute towards our 10 a day, boost our vitamin C levels and may help with conditions like high blood pressure. Smoothies are a good way to add leafy greens to our diet and, when blended with fruit, green vegetables do not seem to have the strong taste that puts some people off. Some researchers argue that when we blend or juice fruit, we're breaking down the plant cell walls and exposing the natural sugars within. Others say that smoothies are a good way for people to nourish themselves and add what they are missing. The best, most healthful smoothies contain about 75% raw rocket / arugula or kale or spinach or Swiss chard and 25% fruit such as banana, mango, citrus, berries or pineapple, with a sprinkle of flax or chia seeds.

*Green Juice or Smoothie Suggestions		
Main ingredients	Kale or spinach or rocket or Bok-choy or Swiss chard or collard greens
	Apple or carrots or blueberries
	Lime or lemon or orange
	Cucumber
	Beetroot
Options	Kiwi fruit, plums, pineapple, blackberries, melon, pears, raspberries, mango. Ground flax and chia seeds, ginger, parsley, basil, mint coriander, beet greens, carrot tops, dandelion, lambs quarter.

5) Do NOT smoke or drink alcohol for the duration of the challenge

Begin by looking forward to giving yourself a reward after quitting smoking and drinking for 7-days. (You might work out how much you have saved and take someone out for a treat to celebrate how much better you feel).

Quitting **smoking** is one of the best things you can do for your health. The sooner you stop, the sooner you will notice changes to your body. After 30 minutes your pulse rate and blood pressure will return to normal. After 8 hours your oxygen levels recover and you have half the amount of harmful carbon monoxide in your blood. After a day your breath and sweat does not smell as bad. Within 48 hours all carbon monoxide is flushed out, your lungs are clearing out mucus and your senses of taste and smell are improving. After 72 hours you will notice that you have more energy and your breathing is easier because your bronchial tubes have started to relax. You start to feel more cheerful and positive. After 2 to 12 weeks you start to look and feel younger, your blood will be pumping through to your heart and muscles much better because your circulation will have improved. After 3 to 9 months any coughs, wheezes or breathing problems will be much better as your lung function increases by up to 10%. After 1 year your risk of heart attack will have halved and after 10 smoke-free years, you're no more likely to die of lung cancer than someone who never smoked. Start today, make a plan and tell a friend or partner that, for the next 7-days (at least), you will not smoke, they can support and hold you to that promise. Use distractions and alternatives if need be, such as dancing and carrots. There are also quit-smoking classes, apps, counselling, medication, and hypnosis.

Stacks of research prove that long tern consumption of **alcohol** has harmful effects on our well-being and many of our organs. Our health improves when we stop or reduce the amount of alcohol we consume, especially if we have a habit of binge drinking. Our skin looks younger, our heart health improves, our immune function gets better, we sleep more deeply and our cancer risk decreases. Giving it up for a week gives us a sense of accomplishment and control over our life. That said, if you depend on alcohol, it may be important to ask for advice before quitting.

It takes 6 to 72 hours for alcohol to leave your system. Within 4 days you should feel more hydrated, less fatigued and start to sleep better. Alcohol may help you fall asleep faster because it is a depressant, but it prevents the all-important REM stage of sleep. Alcohol is a diuretic, it flushes out fluids, so you will feel more hydrated when you consume less, which could improve your oral and skin health. If alcohol was triggering skin conditions, like rosacea, dandruff, psoriasis, or eczema, you could see them begin to improve within a week. After 2 weeks your stomach lining has had time to heal from constant attack and inflammation and returns to normal. You have probably reduced your intake of calories so may start to lose weight. By 3 weeks most drinkers have reduced their high cholesterol and high blood pressure, improved their kidney and eye health and lowered their risk of heart disease and stroke. Your liver is able to devote more time to help your body detox and its other 500 vital functions. After 1 month of not drinking, your liver fat may be reduced by up to 20%, significantly reducing your risk of cirrhosis of the liver or fatty liver disease. 3 months of not drinking reduces your risk of liver, oral, breast, pharynx, larynx, oesophagus, stomach, colorectal and ovarian cancers. When your dopamine levels return to normal, and your mood improves, you find more joy in experiences, people, and situations and your relationships improve.

6) Be a good example

Show good manners. Smile and be friendly, sincere and patient. Treat people the way you would like to be treated. Take responsibility and take pride in doing your best. Look after other people, be kind and do good deeds without expecting to be paid back. Stand up for what's right. Do something nice every day. Acts of kindness make the world a happier place for everyone. They boost feelings of confidence, being in control, pleasure and optimism, and encourage others to do good deeds and contribute to a more positive community. Being kind gives us rewards in many ways from reducing anxiety to living longer. Research shows that people derive satisfaction from helping others, experience fewer aches and pains and live longer. Kindness can keep you young at heart by stimulating the release of oxytocin and nitric oxide, both of which protect the heart by expanding blood vessels and lowering blood pressure.

7) Nurture Relationships

Good relationships are key to physical and mental well-being, they make us happy and keep us healthy. Our social life is a living system which needs maintenance. We should listen, connect and communicate. Forgive, share and persevere. To have healthy relationship people need to make efforts, put in time, give attention, and show love. Social factors have a dramatic effect on our health. Research studies point to the importance of not feeling isolated or lonely and being treated with respect and courtesy.

Stress is a natural part of life. When it happens, our body goes into fight-or-flight mode, our heart rate increases, our blood pressure goes up, we prepare to meet a challenge. If we have someone to talk to when we are stressed or upset, we become calmer. If not, we develop higher levels of circulating stress hormones and higher levels of inflammation, which gradually wear away our systems. We evolved to be social creatures; many people find that being alone is stressful. Good relationships protect our health.

8) Joy and Enjoy

Joy and enjoyment are two closely related emotions. Joy is a feeling of deep pleasure or happiness that comes from within. It is a state of mind that is often associated with positive experiences, accomplishments, or relationships. Joy can be experienced as a result of a personal achievement or a moment of deep connection with someone else. It has been described as a sense of euphoria that fills the heart with warmth and positivity.

Enjoyment, on the other hand, is the act of taking pleasure in an activity, experience, circumstance or environment. It is a more active emotion that involves engaging with something that brings delight or satisfaction. Enjoyment can be experienced in a wide range of activities, such as playing a sport, or listening to music, or spending time in nature or with friends and family.

Both joy and enjoyment are important for overall well-being. Joy can help to create a sense of purpose and meaning in life, while enjoyment provides a sense of contentment, fulfilment and satisfaction in daily activities. They can work together, with the experience of enjoyment leading to feelings of joy and happiness.

It is important to prioritize joy and enjoyment in our lives, as they can help to reduce stress and improve mental health. This can be achieved by being positive, (not negative), engaging in activities that bring us pleasure and satisfaction, such as hobbies, spending time with loved ones, or exploring new experiences. By cultivating joy and enjoyment, we can lead happier, more fulfilling lives.

Your Follow Up Assessment

After following these guidelines for 7-days, go back and do the assessments again (Mind, Body, Exercise, Nutrition and the Central Issues) and see what differences there are. Where did you score better? Any negatives? What is your new *More From Life* score?

Your Second More From Life Score = (/500)

Chapter 9

The 7-Week Challenge and the 7-Month Challenge

Now that you have completed **the One Week Challenge** would you like to continue on this path or journey towards better health and well-being? If so it is time to look forward to the future and see what else you can achieve. You can continue to test yourself, using the *More From Life* assessments, to find out how you are progressing and to build your score closer to 500. You may also start to notice changes such as feeling happier, more attractive, positive, confident and in better shape, being less moody, getting stronger, having more energy and stamina, replacing fat with muscle and getting fewer illnesses and injuries.

What would you like to achieve?

You may enjoy and benefit from setting yourself new goals and targets to see what you can achieve in 7 weeks and then in 7 months. For example, would you like to lose some weight? If so set yourself a reasonable weight loss amount and check your progress every week. You can track and update your BMI, waist to height and body fat scores. Take photos of yourself at the beginning of these challenges so that you can compare before and after.

You might like to make a commitment to change bad habits or attend a gym regularly or go on ParkRuns. Talk to a dietician and a personal trainer about what you are doing and see what they advise. Look at this list of *More From Life* objectives and tick all the ones that you like and want to achieve. Add a time scale so that you can look back at the list in 7 weeks and 7 months to see what you accomplished.

More From Life Objectives. What you want to achieve in 7 weeks and or 7 months? Tick all that apply.	
Reduce stress and feel calmer	
Practice meditation / mindfulness more often	
Feel more fulfilled, happy and content	
Become more confident and empowered	
Get more out of life	
Adjust your work / life balance	
Change your job	
Start a new business or project	
Take part in a charity event	
Volunteer and do community work	
Connect more with friends and family	
Be a better parent to your children / grandchildren	
Improve and grow your social circle	
Explore romantic relationships	
Get ready to get married	
Go on a challenging quest or spectacular holiday	
Learn a new language or skill	
Track and improve your nutrition	
Adopt a more ethical & environmentally friendly diet	
Become a vegetarian or flexitarian or vegan	
Learn to cook better / healthier meals	
Grow your own vegetables	
Spend more time in the garden / in nature	
Write a book or blog, or paint or make videos	
Lose some weight	
Get rid of belly fat	
Gain some weight	
Try intermittent fasting	

More From Life Objectives. What you want to achieve in 7 weeks and or 7 months? Tick all that apply.	
Cut out smoking, cut down on alcohol / drugs	
Get fitter and stronger	
Get advice from a personal trainer or dietician	
Improve your personal best	
Go dancing and or get dancing lessons	
Do more cycling, mountain biking or swimming	
Play more golf or table tennis or football	
Run a marathon or half-marathon or triathlon	
Go hill walking and climb mountains	
Prepare to take up a sport your used to play / do	
Try a totally new sport (eg surfing or roller skating)	
Do strength / weight / resistance training	
Develop your physique / your beach body	
Become more flexible and agile	
Go for saunas / cold-water therapy	
Have a massage or reflexology session	
Make appointment with dentist and or optician	
Get a medical check up	
Help friends and relatives become healthier	
Try to prevent, deal with, arrest or possibly reverse chronic disease such as diabetes, heart disease, and some cancers.	
Other:	

To begin with it may be helpful to write one of your challenges or ambitions down in the middle of a large sheet of paper. Surround this sentence or phrase with the words and ideas that come to mind as you think about it. Let yourself be prompted by questions like:

- Why is this important to me?
- How will I achieve this?

- What stages will it go through?
- What preparations are required?
- Do I need to contact anyone?
- Who will be involved and who do I want to help me accomplish this?
- Where will it happen?
- What do I need to find out about and learn?
- How long will it take?
- How much will it cost?
- What will motivate and keep me going?
- When can I start?
- Do I need any special equipment or resources?
- What health and well-being benefits do I expect from this?
- How will I measure progress and achievement?

You should be able to cover the page with ideas surprisingly quickly. Use these ideas to map out a schedule. Follow this technique with each ambition or objective and it will not take long to develop a comprehensive action plan.

Considerations

Having read this book, had a go at the assessments and recorded many measurements, you will have a wide and reasonably comprehensive range of scores, results, markers and indicators to use as starting points to look back on. You can continue to monitor these as time goes by. Even if you take time off, you can always return to them.

Your body wants to be healthy and heal itself. It has a remarkable capacity to look after us, fix whatever is going wrong and deal with the damage we cause it, if and when we give it a chance and address underlying problems. Many of the quick-fix potions and medicines people take tackle symptoms not causes. It's a bit like continually scratching and picking off the scab that forms over a wound, instead of allowing it to heal, or fixing countless punctures instead of picking up all the nails that are scattered on the ground, or mopping up the floor whenever it rains instead of fixing the roof. Smoking is a good example – smokers often develop coughs and sore throats but, instead of quitting, they buy throat sweets. People with heart disease may end up having angina, heart attacks, strokes, stents, bypasses and even transplants instead of adopting a healthy lifestyle and diet.

Obesity, diabetes and heart disease are becoming so common we are getting used to them, as if they are natural and normal. They are not. Evidence shows that they can be delayed and prevented in almost every case by making sufficient changes in diet and lifestyle.

The suggestions mentioned in this book are inexpensive, within most people's reach and effective. Research shows that many people with high blood pressure, coronary heart disease, diabetes and high cholesterol levels have been able (with the agreement and supervision of their doctor) to reduce and in some cases discontinue, their medications when they make appropriate changes to their lifestyle and diet.

Of course, Lifestyle Medicine is a huge subject covering a wealth of issues and the *More From Life* approach does not address all of the topics that might be considered important and beneficial. The final parts of this book discuss some of these factors and considerations.

Stress, Contentment and Fulfilment

Stress can cause many problems including headaches, tension, fear, anger, hostility, depression, insomnia, road rage, anxiety, ulcers, high blood pressure, dissatisfaction, sexual impotence and inability to concentrate. It can affect our immune system. We need to figure out where our stress comes from and do what we can to reduce and deal with those factors and influences. How we feel about ourselves and how we relate to other people are very important. Research suggests that these aspects of our lives are vital to our health and well-being.

- Take care of yourself.
- Relax and release.
- Spend time each day giving yourself some peace and quiet. Take time out. Calm down and allow distracting thoughts to drift away like hot air balloons. Access the "Headspace" app and follow the advice.

- Join teams, organisations and groups and connect with others, especially if you feel lonely and isolated.

- Make an effort to be kind. It can feel good to develop a habit of being nice and helping others. Try to take opportunities to be altruistic, empathetic, compassionate and supportive whenever you can.

- Look after relationships. Spend lots of time with your friends, family and communities. Invite them for meals, or to go bowling or for walks together.

- Get plenty of exercise.

- Do things you feel good about – things to be proud of.

- Have a sense of purpose. Decide what is important. Make plans and stick to them. Set yourself targets and goals. Measure your progress, monitor and learn from your setbacks and celebrate your successes.

Green spaces, spending time in nature

We are beginning to understand how important access to outdoor natural space is for our mental and physical well-being. The number of people living in cities is booming. By 2050, projections suggest almost 70 per cent of us will be urban dwellers. Evidence of positive effects from nature includes studies on psychological conditions such as depression, anxiety and mood disorders. Access to nature has been found to improve sleep and reduce stress, increase happiness and reduce negative emotions, promote positive social interactions and even help generate a sense of meaning to life. Being in green environments boosts various aspects of thinking, including attention, memory and creativity. Some doctors have begun to prescribe nature-based activities such as gardening, "forest bathing", birdwatching and beach walks to treat mental health conditions and stress, as well as physical conditions such as heart disease and diabetes.

Breathwork

Breathwork and deep abdominal breathing are exercises or techniques that can improve mental, physical, and spiritual well-being which many people find promote deep relaxation and / or give them energy. People have been practicing breathwork for thousands of years. The basic idea is to nourish your mind and body with oxygen when you breathe in and release toxins and stress when you breathe out. You change your usual (shallow) breathing routine by taking a set of 5 to 30 long deep breaths, fill your lungs with each breath, rest for a minute and do that set again. Do this for 5 to 10 minutes. As you breathe, you visualize your breath filling up your body. Your belly and chest should expand when you inhale and you expel most of this air when you exhale. You can if you like try the 5-6-7 breathing pattern, in which you follow a cycle of inhaling deeply through your nose for five seconds, holding your breath for six seconds, and exhaling through your mouth for seven seconds.

Weight Loss

If you are overweight you might like to:

- decrease your sugar, fructose, fizzy drinks, cakes, cheese, yogurt with added sweetener, oil and saturated fat intake.
- Instead eat more vegetables.
- Try intermittent fasting, such as the 5:2 diet (eating normally 5 days a week and reducing your consumption to about 1,000 calories for 2 days a week),
- Restrict your eating time window to about 10 hours, (say 11am to 7pm), to allow the body 14 hours to repair and recover.
- Preload with water, or a green salad, or soup or an apple before a meal.
- Flavour meals and salads with vinegar.
- Take your time. Don't swallow too quickly. Chew food well and extend meal times.
- Stay active.
- Try adding a pinch or two of spices and herbs to your diet such as black cumin, garlic powder, cumin, ginger, nutritional or brewer's or baker's yeast. All have been shown to help with nutrition and weight reduction.

Studies show that calorie counting diets do not work. 1) It is remarkably difficult to count all the calories we eat accurately, 2) we all have different metabolisms, 3) calorie counting treats all calories as if they are of equal value and 4) in the long run, more than 90% of people will go back to their baseline weight (or past it).

Some products contain far more calories than others. Take salads, sugary fizzy drinks, and olive oil as 3 examples. A 240 calorie salad (containing lettuce, tomatoes, carrots, spinach, green snap beans, broccoli, cucumber and celery with some lemon juice, blueberries, raspberries and strawberries), would overflow a plate, take a long time to consume and (more than) fill your stomach, whereas a 240 calorie (20 oz or 590 ml) bottle of sugary pop liquid can be swallowed in minutes and just 2 tablespoons of oil is equal to 240 calories. A basic hamburger from a typical high street outlet (without cheese) is about 260 calories, and one 12 inch cheese pizza can have 1700 calories. So you can probably eat as much salad as you like – feel full without counting calories - and lose weight, but consuming sugary drinks and cakes, fatty hamburgers and pizzas, and oily / processed foods will pour extra calories into you, do you harm and may still leave you feeling hungry. (lettuce = 11 cal / 100g, tomato = 18cal / 100g, cucumber and celery = 15cal / 100g, carrots = 36cal/100g, spinach = 23cal / 100g, green snap beans = 34cal / 100g, olive oil = 880 cal / 100g). So calorie counting may not be the best strategy for losing weight.

Fasting

We are well-adapted to quite prolonged fasting. In prehistoric times, before humans learned to farm, they were daily gatherers and occasional successful hunters. It has been suggested that we are not built to eat three meals a day, every day. Our distant ancestors may have been more likely to eat when they found food and they may have had to survive several days at a time without food. It is argued therefore that fasting is natural and is good for us. We can store large amounts of calories when food is available and this ability to put on weight has led to modern diseases like obesity and type 2 diabetes. Caloric restriction is thought by some to be a fountain of youth.

Therapeutic fasting has been recommended for treating obesity, hypertension, type 2 diabetes, lupus, metabolic disorder, rheumatoid arthritis, depression, anxiety and some skin conditions. While there may be numerous potential health and longevity benefits, negative symptoms can include over-lowering of blood pressure, loss of strength, slower wound healing, loss of libido, menstrual irregularities, infertility, depression and irritability.

Fasting may be a useful way to make a change and begin a new way of eating but it can be difficult to sustain. You can use fasting occasionally or as a kick start to transition to a healthy, whole-food, plant-based diet. Those people who stick to plant-based diets seem to have more long-term success at not putting the weight back on.

Intermittent fasting has become popular recently. It is the practice of abstaining from food for short periods of time, rather than trying to restrict the total amount of calories you consume.

Rather than cutting calories every day, you could try eating as much as you want every other day, or for only a few hours a day. Or you might experiment with fasting two days a week or five days a month. Research studies show that, while there may be certain advantages in these strategies, there are drawbacks also. It may be dangerous to give up eating for longer than 24 hours. In some cases, fasting for 3 days or more should be done under the supervision of a doctor and may require patients to attend a clinic. To be safe you should try to keep your calorie intake above 1,000 a day, even on fasting days. You should not fast if you are diabetic or underweight or have kidney or liver failure or have an active infection or have a history of fainting or are on certain medications or are pregnant or breastfeeding.

Several studies on intermittent fasting show impressive health benefits. It seems to be easier to follow than continuous calorie restriction, reduces body fat and triglycerides and may reduce insulin levels significantly. The 5:2 diet (in which you eat normally for 5 days a week and restrict calorie intake to less than 1000 per day for the other 2) has become a popular intermittent fasting diet. Another approach is to limit the eating window to 8 or 10 hours a day, just drinking water, tea, coffee and or vegetable juice for the other 16 or 14. Fasting may also support motivation for lifestyle change.

Walking

Illnesses caused by our increasingly mechanised vehicle and screen dependant; sedentary, urban lifestyles are becoming epidemics. Too many people, these days, spend their lives indoors, (at home and in the office, car, shopping mall, gym, cinema, café, pub and restaurant), disconnected from nature and natural light, walking just enough to get from one of these spaces to the next. A study that tracked 1,000 adults during flu season found that those who walked for 30 to 45 minutes a day had 43% fewer sick days. Researchers investigating the connection between daily step count, intensity of steps and health benefit have found that walking at a brisk pace (80 steps per minute) and taking 10,000 steps a day, lowers our risk of dementia, cardiovascular disease, cancer and premature death.

Humans are good at walking; we have been bipedal for at least a million years. We are, in many ways, designed to walk. Walking does not require expensive equipment and has numerous health benefits, including reducing excess body fat, improving heart health, strengthening bones and muscles, boosting the immune system, and lifting our spirits. Walking is good for the soul. Walking gives us time to think. The mind works well at walking speed. Walking in a wood, up a hill or mountain, beside a river or the sea, through a valley or along a cliff path, helps us to explore our mental landscape and journey of thoughts. The mind and body work together, thinking and travelling. Rambling encourages a mixture of daydreaming and planning, of memories and futures. This explains why we often have new ideas and insights while walking and why so many walkers carry and write diaries, blogs and journals. Wandering unhurried, along the ups and downs, twists and turns of a track, listening to birds, watching the clouds, smelling the fragrances, feeling the sunlight, shade, breeze, raindrops and seasons, noticing the magnificence and details of trees and flowers, enjoying the rhythm of our footsteps and being part of the landscape. Walking is good for us in so many ways.

Strength training

Walking is good for us but we need to look after all of our muscles, bones, lean tissue, ligaments and tendons. Resistive and strength training is crucial to maintain and restore muscle tone, flexibility and function. We should incorporate strength training into our schedules and devote enough time to it, especially as we get older. Even quite small amounts of strength training can help to slow muscle loss. More muscle means you burn more fat and calories. Strength training also improves bone density, and functional movement. It increases our self-confidence, gives us better balance and symmetry and helps to prevent injury. It can improve our mood, ease symptoms of arthritis, reduce blood pressure and cholesterol, make us feel younger and help us benefit from better sleep. It does not require expensive equipment and can be done at home and outdoors.

Warm up by stretching and dancing or jogging on the spot, then repeat the following set of exercises 3 times:

- do as many push-ups as you can achieve comfortably,

- rotations – take something reasonably large but not too heavy (such as a big cushion from the sofa) and hold it out in front of you, keeping your feet still and your arms horizontal and straight, rotate your upper body so that the object moves from your left side to your right and back again. Do this 10 times.

- Lie on your back on the floor and lift one leg ten times then do the same with the other,

- hold a plank position as long as you can,

- do 10 dips – put your hands behind you on the edge of the seat of a kitchen or dining chair and lower your bottom towards the floor then use the strength in your arms to push back up,

- sit normally on the edge of this chair and then stand up. Repeat this squatting motion as often as you can, dropping your bottom down so that it touches the chair then pushing back up, your quads should start to burn.

- do as many burpees as you can, they strengthen the muscles in your legs, hips, buttocks, abdomen, arms, chest, and shoulders. Do a press up to start, then bring your knees up to your chin, stand and jump up, pointing your hands to the sky before dropping back to a press-up position, and repeating the movement.

- bicep curls – bend your arms at the elbow while lifting a weight in each hand – choose weights that you are able to lift

8 to 15 times, for example fill a shopping bag with tins if you do not have dumbbells or kettlebell/s.

Take it slow to begin with, get your doctor's ok if need be. Stop if you feel pain. You could spend about 30 minutes to an hour every 2 or 3 days doing strength training exercises, your muscles will need about 48 hours rest before the next workout.

HIIT

HIIT (High-intensity interval training) is a broad term for workouts that involve short periods of intense exercise alternated with recovery periods. It involves repeated, quick, anaerobic, explosive bursts of action performed at maximum or near maximal effort levels, (to the point of exhaustion), with brief periods of rest between bouts. A typical HIIT burst might last 20 to 40 seconds. For example, an HIIT workout using a stationary bike could consist of 30 seconds of cycling as fast as possible with high resistance, followed by a period of slow, easy cycling with low resistance. This would be considered one rep, and you would expect to complete 4–6 reps in one workout. Alternatively, you could also use battle-ropes or elliptical trainers. HIIT is said to provide a range of health benefits. It can burn a lot of calories in a short amount of time; reduce heart rate, blood sugar and blood pressure; improve oxygen consumption; help you lose fat; increase muscle mass; and raise your metabolic rate for hours after the workout.

Yoga and Pilates

Yoga is a set of posture-related fitness, stress-relief and relaxation practices and techniques that began as a group of physical, mental, and spiritual disciplines in ancient India.

Pilates was invented as way to help dancers through injury, it is a type of exercise in which you perform a series of controlled movements that flow into one another with precision. It balances your muscles by targeting and strengthening the ones you do not often use in your daily life.

Yoga focuses on mobility and stretching, while Pilates emphasizes building functional strength. Some people find they enjoy and benefit from regular Yoga and or Pilates sessions. If you have never tried, it might be worth giving them a try. Classes are usually available in most towns and many gyms. If you are new to yoga or Pilates you could attend a beginner's class or watch and try a beginner's video. If you have already sampled Yoga or Pilates, is it time to go back and give it another go?

Chapter 10

Interesting Foods, Nutrients, Spices and Herbs

While the key ingredients of nutrition (discussed in chapter 6) include: fibre, antioxidants, alkaline-forming foods, electrolytes, phytonutrients, essential fats, iron, calcium, protein, carbohydrates, vitamins and minerals, all of which are found in abundance in plant-based nutrition, there are some specifics that are worth mentioning.

Beetroot are colourful root vegetables that are packed with essential nutrients, vitamins, minerals, and plant compounds, many of which have medicinal properties. Beetroots are a great source of fibre, folate (vitamin B9), manganese, copper, potassium, iron, vitamin C and vitamin B6. They have been associated with numerous health benefits, including improved blood flow, lower blood pressure, and increased exercise performance. Studies show that beetroot juice's high concentration of nitrates can lower levels of both systolic and diastolic blood pressure significantly. Dietary nitrates are converted into nitric oxide, a molecule that dilates blood vessels.

Amla, also known as the Indian gooseberry, is one of the most antioxidant-rich foods on Earth and has been called a wonder berry for treating cancer. It seems to block cancer cell invasion and cancer growth. Indian gooseberries have been found to have cholesterol-lowering as well as fever, pain, stress, diarrhea, cough and stress suppressing effects. Recent research suggests that it may also work as a diabetes drug.

Nutritional yeast is a seasoning that offers a savoury or umami flavour. It is often used in vegan cooking as a substitute for cheese. Nutritional yeast is a good source of plant-based protein, B vitamins, trace minerals and two teaspoons of nutritional yeast packs over 300% of the recommended daily amount for vitamin B12.

Honey. People all over the world love honey for its sweetness and depth of flavour and it is used in many recipes. Honey has no fat and only trace amounts of protein and fibre, it contains small amounts of some nutrients and is rich in health-promoting antioxidants and compounds known as polyphenols. It is thought to offer antidepressant, anticonvulsant and anti-anxiety benefits. The smell, colour and taste of honey vary depending on the type of flowers the bees visited. Raw honey has been used as a remedy throughout history and has a variety of health benefits and medical uses. Most of the honey in supermarkets is pasteurized. The high heat kills unwanted yeast, can improve the colour and texture, removes any crystallization, and extends the shelf life, however, many of the beneficial nutrients are destroyed in the process. The topical use of medical-grade honey has been shown to promote wound healing, particularly in burns.

Maple syrup is another sweetener that is used in some recipes. It could be described as a less bad version of sugar. Replacing refined sugar with good quality maple syrup may yield a marginal net health benefit, but it is best to add it in moderation.

Sugar. Many people eat far too much refined and added sugar. On average, adults consume the equivalent of 24 teaspoons of sugar (almost 400 calories) per day. It is in so many foods nowadays that it is difficult to avoid and we need to read ingredient labels carefully when buying packaged / man-made food products. Typical sources include: soft drinks, fruit drinks, flavoured yogurts, cereals, biscuits, cakes, sweets, many soups, bread, cured meats, ketchup and most processed foods. We have already noted that adding sugar can raise blood pressure and cause inflammation, weight gain and fatty liver disease. Research studies (including one that identified 73 meta-analyses from 8601 unique articles), show that high sugar intake contributes to cardiovascular disease, cancers, type 2 diabetes, gout, obesity, tooth decay and other conditions. We should limit our daily sugar intake to about 6 teaspoons (25 grams). Sugar occurs naturally in fruit, vegetables, and grains and eating whole foods that contain natural sugar seems to be okay because we digest these foods slowly. Plant foods have high amounts of fibre, essential minerals, and antioxidants and the sugar in them provides a steady supply of energy to our cells.

Vinegar contains polyphenols, plant chemicals that have an antioxidant effect that may protect cells from oxidative stress, a possible stimulator of tumour growth. To make vinegar, a sugar source such as fruit or grains is fermented and turned into alcohol, then the liquid is fermented again, which converts the alcohol into acid. It has proved to be somewhat effective in helping to lower cholesterol, improve circulation and stabilise blood pressure. Some studies have suggested that vinegar may slow the growth of cancer cells. Balsamic vinegar is a very dark, concentrated and intensely flavoured vinegar made from grapes, it can liven up a salad. Balsamic vinegars may be aged in barrels for months or even years. The active compound in balsamic vinegar is acetic acid, which contains strains of probiotics that aid digestion. Apple cider vinegar can help to manage or control blood sugar spikes after meals rich in carbohydrates, reduce cholesterol levels, lessen inflammation, improve symptoms of polycystic ovary syndrome and promote weight loss. Apple Cider Vinegar may also help to detoxify the liver and flush out harmful toxins. The recommended dose is 1 to 2 tablespoons, (15 to 30 mL) taken before or after meals.

Tamari and soy sauce are both made from fermented soy beans, but tamari contains much less salt than traditional soy sauce. It aids in the digestion of fruits and vegetables, while being rich in several minerals, and is a good source of vitamin B3, protein and manganese. In traditional Chinese medicine, the soybeans from which tamari is derived are thought to have cooling properties and are believed to enhance detoxification, promote regularity and ease urination.

Marmite is a thick, dark-coloured, paste made from the yeast by-product left over from beer brewing with a flavour that is difficult to describe. It was discovered by accident when a scientist realised that left-over brewer's yeast could be concentrated and eaten. The first Marmite production was established in 1902 in Burton on Trent in the UK and since then it has become the quintessential "love it or hate it" product.

People eat it with toast and in stews and sauces. Research into Marmite's health benefits shows that it is a source of several vitamins and minerals, including: Vitamin B6, Vitamin B12, Potassium, Magnesium, Thiamine, Riboflavin, Niacin and Folate. However it is so salty that a 10 gram serving packs 330mg of sodium, which is around 14% of your daily recommended amount

Fermented foods may offer a range of health benefits. Fermentation is an ancient technique for preserving food and drinks, produced by controlled microbial growth and enzyme actions, which convert some of the food into other compounds. Fermented foods are an important part of the diet in many cultures and fermentation has been associated with a range of health benefits. Fermented foods are a source of probiotics.

Microorganisms, like bacteria, yeast and fungi, convert organic compounds, like sugars and starch, into alcohol or acids. These act as natural preservatives and produce a distinctive strong, salty and slightly sour flavour. Microorganisms such as lactic acid bacteria (LAB) have been studied for their effects. They are said to have anti-carcinogenic, anti-microbial, anti-oxidant, anti-allergenic, anti-diabetic and anti-atherosclerotic properties and to lower blood pressure.

Common fermented foods include: certain aged cheeses with active cultures, plain yogurt, kefir, dry curd cottage cheese, sauerkraut, fermented vegetables, tempeh, miso, pickles (in salt, not vinegar), natto, apple cider, kimchi and kombucha.

Sauerkraut, (sour cabbage) is finely-cut, fermented, raw cabbage with many health benefits including boosting the immune system. It has a long shelf life and a distinctive sour flavour which come from the lactic acid formed when bacteria ferment the sugars in the cabbage leaves. The fermentation process increases the bioavailability of nutrients. It is high in vitamins K and C and it is a good source of fibre, folate, iron, potassium, copper, sodium manganese, calcium and magnesium. The fibre and probiotics improve digestion and promote the growth of healthy bowel flora, protecting against many diseases of the digestive tract.

Kombucha is a fermented, slightly effervescent, sweetened black tea drink commonly consumed for its health benefits. Sometimes the beverage is called kombucha tea to distinguish it from the culture of bacteria and yeast. Juices, spices, fruit or other flavourings are often added.

Kimchi is a Korean side dish of salted and fermented vegetables, that may be eaten with almost every meal. Many types of kimchi are made using different vegetables as the main ingredients, with a range of seasonings, including spring onions, garlic, ginger, and salted seafood. Kimchi is also used in soups and stews.

Vitamin B12 plays an essential role in red blood cell formation, cell metabolism, nerve function and the production of DNA. Since our body does not make vitamin B12, many people need to get it from regular supplements. While B12 is stored in the liver for up to five years, we can eventually become deficient. The symptoms of a vitamin B12 deficiency may include: pale yellow tinge to one's skin, sore and red tongue, mouth ulcers, heart palpitations, pins and needles, disturbed vision, irritability, depression, changes in behaviour and thinking, decline in mental abilities including memory and judgement, changes in mobility.

Vitamin C is important for wound healing, keeping the cells in our skin, bones, cartilage and blood healthy, boosting immunity and may help to protect us against gout. In rare cases lack of vitamin C can lead to scurvy. Also known as ascorbic acid, Vitamin C is found in a wide variety of fruit and vegetables including: oranges, lemons, bell peppers, strawberries, cabbage, blackcurrants, broccoli, kale, potatoes and Brussel sprouts. Vitamin C cannot be stored in the body, we need it in our diet every day, but we should be able to get all the vitamin C we need from our wholefood balanced diet.

Vitamin D helps to keep our bones, teeth and muscles healthy. It can reduce cancer cell growth; help control infections and reduce inflammation. There is evidence that people who take Vitamin D have 40% lower risk of dementia. It may also reduce the chance of developing diabetes. The body creates vitamin D from direct sunlight on the skin. Most people should be able to make all the vitamin D they need from sunlight in summer, but many of us may not make enough between October and March. For that reason, government advice suggests that everyone should think about taking a vitamin D supplement regularly during the autumn and winter. We should try to spend some time outdoors every day. We cannot overdose on vitamin D through exposure to sunshine, but we need to cover up or protect our skin, if we spend long periods outside in strong sunlight, to reduce the risk of skin damage and skin cancer.

Omega-3 Fatty Acids. The two main types of fatty acids are saturated and unsaturated (polyunsaturated and monounsaturated fat). Saturated fats have been named "bad" fats because they increase our risk of heart disease and stroke.

Omega-3 fatty acids, on the other hand, are polyunsaturated fats that have potential benefits. They are essential nutrients sometimes called "healthy fats" because they can reduce our triglyceride levels and may help to raise our HDL (good) cholesterol, improve circulation and lower our blood pressure. Some studies have shown omega-3s may reduce our risk for: cardiovascular disease, blood clots, rheumatoid arthritis, some forms of cancer, age-related macular degeneration, depression, dementia and Alzheimer's disease.

Specific types of omega-3s include DHA and EPA (found in seafood) and ALA (found in plants). Some foods that can help us add omega-3s to our diet include: algae, walnuts, edamame, and pumpkin, flax and chia seeds. Oily fish such as salmon, mackerel and sardines are often recommended but fish oil may be so contaminated with PCBs, dioxins and other pollutants that a person's overall daily intake may exceed the tolerable limit of toxicity. Omega-3 supplements, such as fish oil pills, can cause side effects and interfere with prescribed medicines. Overall, clinical trials on the benefits of omega-3 supplements have mixed results.

Sulforaphane has been linked to improved heart health and digestion. It is a natural plant compound found in many cruciferous vegetables such as broccoli, cabbage, bok choy, cauliflower, and kale. The beneficial enzymes are released and activated when the plant is damaged, so these vegetables need to be chewed, cut or chopped. Raw cruciferous vegetables have the highest levels of sulforaphane, studies indicate that raw broccoli has ten times more sulforaphane than cooked broccoli.

Nitric Oxide (NO), recent research has led minor revolutions in studies of physiology and pharmacology. NO was proclaimed the "Molecule of the Year" in 1992 and the 1998 Nobel Prize in Physiology or Medicine was awarded for discovering nitric oxide's role as a cardiovascular signalling molecule. Nitric oxide production is essential for overall health because it allows blood, nutrients, and oxygen to travel to every part of our body effectively and efficiently. It relaxes blood vessels, causing them to widen and increase circulation. A limited capacity to produce nitric oxide is associated with heart disease, diabetes, and erectile dysfunction.

Nitric oxide is an unstable molecule that degrades quickly in the bloodstream, so it must be constantly replenished, this can be done by consuming antioxidants. Good sources of nitrate and antioxidant rich food include dark green leafy vegetables like kale, arugula, Swiss Chard, spinach, beets, cabbage, cauliflower, carrots and broccoli. Studies have shown that eating nitrate-rich vegetables can lower blood pressure as much as some blood pressure medications and there is strong evidence in favour of nitrates, especially from beetroot, for improving exercise performance in athletes. (Nitrates in processed meats, however, can be troublesome to health, particularly when consumed in excess over long periods).

Certain bacteria in our mouths convert nitrate to nitric oxide. Humans use these bacteria to produce nitric oxide. Mouthwash kills bacteria, including the beneficial ones that help generate nitric oxide. The detrimental effects of mouthwash on nitric oxide production may even contribute to the development of diabetes. One study found that people who used mouthwash twice daily were 49% more likely to develop diabetes than those who never used mouthwash.

The thin layer of cells that line blood vessels are known as endothelial cells. These cells help to keep much of the cardiovascular system healthy. Insufficient nitric oxide production results in endothelium dysfunction, which causes atherosclerosis, high blood pressure, and other risk factors for heart disease. Studies have shown that exercise improves endothelial function and improves antioxidant activity, which helps inhibit the breakdown of nitric oxide caused by free radicals. The benefits of exercise on nitric oxide production and endothelial health can be felt in as little as ten weeks, when exercising for 30 minutes at least 3 times a week.

Surprisingly, breathing through the nose and humming are thought to be good ways to help our NO intake. Nasal sinuses are major producers of nitric oxide. The oscillating airflow produced by humming may enhance sinus ventilation and thereby increase nasal NO levels. In a recent study NO increased 15 fold during humming compared with quiet breathing.

Your nose is designed to help you to breathe safely, efficiently, and properly. It can filter out foreign particles like dust, allergens, and pollen and humidify inhaled air. Nose breathing also improves air flow to arteries, veins, and nerves; increases oxygen uptake and circulation; reduces your risk of coughing; aids your immune system and lowers your risk of sleep apnoea and snoring.

Coffee is a very popular beverage. We drink well over a million tons of coffee every year. Population studies suggest that coffee drinkers have lower risk of Parkinson's, and less: prostate and liver cancer, diabetes, liver cirrhosis, depression, and overall mortality. It seems that coffee drinkers tend to live longer than non-coffee drinkers.

In studies, people with Parkinson's and chronic hepatitis, seem to improve within a few weeks when they consume about two cups of coffee's worth of caffeine per day. Runners complete a mile about six seconds quicker and weightlifters can squat more weight, when they drink coffee. It is not certain, however, if coffee consumption makes the difference, those who drink coffee may just happen to exercise more. What is more, people respond differently. While most people metabolize caffeine rapidly, some people are slow metabolizers. Those who have impaired caffeine metabolism genes have an elevated risk of becoming hypertensive and caffeine can spike adrenaline levels in their blood. Conversely, it appears that rapid metabolizers lower their risk of hypertension the more coffee they drink, the beneficial polyphenol antioxidants lower their blood pressure. Even at four or more cups a day, rapid metabolizers can clear caffeine so fast that they feel little increase in adrenaline. Daily coffee consumption, (especially at high levels), seems to multiply the chances of having a heart attack in slow metabolizers, whereas drinking coffee is protective in rapid caffeine metabolizers, cutting their odds of heart attack by more than half. So, consuming coffee may put slow caffeine metabolizers at increased risk of cardiovascular disease, but protect fast caffeine metabolizers.

Garlic (Allium sativum) is a popular, nutritious and powerful herb related to onions, leeks, and chives which is often credited with health benefits for treating conditions related to the cardio vascular system. It has been used by the ancient Babylonians, Egyptians, Greeks, Romans, and Chinese. Hippocrates, the Greek physician born in 460BC, is supposed to have said "Let food be thy medicine, and medicine be thy food." He prescribed garlic to treat a variety of conditions and modern science has confirmed many of these beneficial health effects. Garlic is known to fight common infectious diseases so people with dysfunctional immune systems may benefit from taking it. Garlic contains antioxidants that help the body's protective mechanisms against oxidative damage. High doses of garlic supplements (equivalent to about 6 cloves per day) have been shown to reduce oxidative stress in people with high blood pressure and, in some cases, to be as effective at reducing blood pressure as prescribed blood pressure drugs.

Garlic can reduce total and LDL cholesterol by about 10–15%. The combination of antioxidant properties and reductions in cholesterol and blood pressure, may reduce the risk of common brain conditions like Alzheimer's disease and dementia. There is some evidence that garlic can increase blood flow and nitric oxide levels which helps blood vessels dilate and is a treatment for erectile dysfunction in men. One of the few potential drawbacks is that eating too much garlic may increase the risk of bleeding, especially if one is taking blood thinners or undergoing surgery.

Turmeric (Curcuma longa) is a very effective nutritional supplement which has been used for thousands of years in cooking and medicine. Studies show that it can offer benefits to both the body and the brain. Curcumin, the active compound in turmeric, is a substance with powerful anti-inflammatory and antioxidant properties that can be effective for alleviating a range of conditions. Inflammation plays a role in many illnesses and health problems, including: heart disease, metabolic syndrome, Alzheimer's disease, various degenerative conditions and cancers of the breast, brain, blood, colon, kidney, liver, pancreas, and skin, and may also help speed recovery after surgery. Unlike most chemotherapy drugs, against which cancer cells can develop resistance, curcumin affects several mechanisms of cell death simultaneously, making it potentially harder for cancer cells to avoid destruction. For reasons not fully understood, curcumin seems to leave noncancerous cells alone.

Turmeric is also recommended by some dieticians as a supplement for arthritis, digestive disorders, respiratory infections, allergies, liver disease, depression and anxiety. A multicenter, randomized, placebo-controlled, double-blind study found that more than 50% of ulcerative colitis patients achieved remission within a month on curcumin compared to none of the patients who received the placebo. Turmeric and curcumin supplements are considered safe, but very high doses may lead to diarrhoea, headache, or skin irritation.

Flax seeds are one of the first health foods. Treasured by the ancient Greeks for their healing properties, they are very high in alpha-linolenic acid (ALA) omega-3s. A 100-gram portion of ground flax seed supplies about 2,234 kilojoules (534 kilocalories) of food energy, 41 g of fat, 28 g of fibre, and 20 g of protein. Consumption of 30g of flax-seed per day for 12 weeks has been shown to reduce body weight and waist circumference, reduce many patients' blood pressure, total and LDL-cholesterol and improve blood sugars, triglycerides, cholesterol, and haemoglobin A1c levels in diabetics. Ground flax seeds may work two to three times better than blood pressure medicines and only have good side effects.

Flax seeds appear to reduce human breast cancer risk by 20% to 30% and slow breast tumour growth in just a few weeks. Flaxseeds are packed with lignans, (they have about 100 times more lignans than other foods), only a small daily serving is required to attain the level of lignan intake associated with a reduction in breast cancer risk.

Most men over 50 suffer from an enlarged prostate. They need to get out of bed often at night and may experience sexual dysfunction, prostate cancer and depression. Studies suggest that consuming less, (or no), animal protein (such as eggs and poultry) and increasing the intake of fruits and vegetables may be protective. Cranberries were used by Native Americans to treat urinary ailments, and significant improvements have been seen in prostate problems and quality of life, with just a teaspoon of powdered cranberries per day. Pumpkin seeds also seem to make a difference.

Evidence suggests that ground flax seeds are a safe and inexpensive source of nutrition that have many benefits including reducing tumour proliferation rates.

Black Cumin has been used for centuries to treat everything from abscesses to herpes. It is said to enhance the immune system, protect against cancer and fight inflammation. Some studies suggest that black cumin promotes wound healing and can reduce the severity of skin problems like psoriasis and acne.

Herbal remedies are made with active ingredients derived from plant leaves, roots or flowers and presented in various forms, such as capsules, teas, liquid drops or skin creams. Cultures around the world have relied on traditional herbal medicine to meet their healthcare needs for centuries and the demand for herbal remedies is rising. However it should be noted that most of these "natural" products are not as strictly regulated as conventional medicines.

It is best to consult a specialist or health professional before taking herbal remedies to ensure proper dosage, understand potential side effects, and become aware of potential reactions with other medications. For example: raw elderberries can be toxic, St. John's Wort can interact dangerously with antidepressants, and valerian root can compound the effects of sedatives. Many herbal medicines have not been studied rigorously enough to verify their safety for pregnant or breastfeeding women. In some countries herbal product manufacturers do not have to provide proof of efficacy or purity when they market their merchandise. Some supplements may list ingredients improperly or contain compounds not stated on the label.

Oregano is available fresh, dried and as oil. It can be added to stews and pasta dishes, dressings and sauces. Rich in antioxidants and vitamin K, it is said to have remarkable health giving properties including fighting off viruses and bacteria, reducing inflammation and possibly slowing the growth of cancer cells.

Ginseng roots are usually steeped to make a tea or dried to make a powder. It is used in traditional Chinese medicine to boost immunity, brain function, and energy levels and reduce inflammation but there is little research evidence supporting its efficacy. Some studies have suggested that it has protective, anti-cancer, anti-diabetes, and immune-supporting properties. Short-term use of ginseng is thought to be safe.

Valerian is sometimes referred to as "nature's Valium," because its roots are thought to induce a sense of tranquillity and calm. The root can be dried and used in capsules or steeped to make tea. The use of valerian can be traced back to ancient Greece and Rome, where it was taken to relieve restlessness, tremors, headaches, and heart palpitations. These days it is used by some to treat insomnia and anxiety, although there is little evidence to verify these assumptions. Valerian is considered reasonably safe, it may cause mild side effects like headaches and digestive issues, but one should probably not take it when on other sedatives.

Ginger is often used in cooking and herbal medicine. It has been used to treat colds, migraines, and high blood pressure. There are claims that it can relieve the nausea associated with pregnancy, chemotherapy, and medical operations. It can be eaten fresh or dried and, in a tea, or capsule. Negative side effects are rare, but large doses may cause a mild case of heartburn or diarrhoea.

Elderberry extracts are available as a syrup or lozenge to relieve the symptoms of colds and flu. An ancient herbal medicine, it was used to relieve headaches, nerve pain, toothaches, colds, viral infections, and constipation. Short-term use is considered safe, but elderberry is toxic if eaten raw or unripe and it can cause nausea, vomiting, and diarrhoea.

St. John's wort's use as a herbal medicine can be traced back to ancient Greece. It is still prescribed by health professionals in parts of Europe to aid wound healing and alleviate insomnia, depression, and various kidney and lung diseases. Its small, yellow flowers are commonly used to make teas, capsules, or extracts. Some people believe that using St John's wort for short periods of time can be as effective as conventional antidepressants, but it is not clear if long term use is safe or effective, especially for those who have severe depression or suicidal thoughts. St John's wort seems to have few side effects but may cause allergic reactions, dizziness, confusion, dry mouth, increased light sensitivity and may interfere with conventional medications such as antidepressants, birth control, blood thinners, certain pain medications, and some types of cancer treatments. These interactions can be so severe that, in rare cases, they can be fatal, so it is best to consult a doctor before using it.

Ginkgo is an herbal medicine, derived from the maidenhair tree, that contains a variety of potent antioxidants that are thought to provide several benefits. Ginkgo has been used in traditional Chinese medicine for thousands of years and is still a top-selling herbal supplement today. It is used to treat a wide range of ailments, including heart disease, dementia and sexual dysfunction, but studies have yet to prove that it is effective for any of these conditions. Although well tolerated by most people, possible side effects include headache, heart palpitations, digestive issues, skin reactions, and an increased risk of bleeding.

Echinacea, or coneflower, is a flowering plant and popular herbal tea or supplement used to reduce the risk of getting the common cold. It was also used in North America to treat various ailments, including wounds, burns, toothaches, sore throats, and upset stomachs. Rare side effects might include: nausea, stomach pain, and skin rash.

Chamomile is one of the most popular herbal medicines in the world. The flowers and leaves can be used to make tea, medicinal extracts, or topical compresses. It has been regarded as a remedy for: wounds, nausea, diarrhoea, constipation, stomach pain, cramping, urinary tract infections, arthritis and respiratory infections for hundreds of years. Studies indicate it may have anti-inflammatory, antimicrobial, and antioxidant properties. Chamomile tea is safe for most people but could cause slight allergic reactions.

Hibiscus, also known as **Roselle**, is a nutritious plant used to treat hypertension and to help with nervous system disorders. Hibiscus tea is served both hot and cold. It has many different names in many countries around the world and is well known for its red colour, tartness and unique flavour. Dried hibiscus is edible and it can be used as a garnish. Modern research appears to confirm that hibiscus can lower blood pressure, balance blood lipids, support liver health, and aid weight loss. Hibiscus seems to be a safe and well-tolerated herb.

Rooibos is a fragrant, caffeine-free tea, made from the leaves and stems of the Aspalathus linearis tree, which grows in South Africa, where rooibos tea is a national drink. Rooibos is associated with health benefits due to its high levels of health-promoting antioxidants which help protect cells from damage by free radicals. There are claims that It can help to prevent cancer, heart disease, indigestion and hay fever, but there is little credible scientific evidence to support these views. Rooibos seems to have very few side effects.

Peppermint tea and oil have been found to be effective at relieving symptoms of irritable bowel syndrome and the digestive discomfort caused by cramping, nausea or indigestion. Evidence shows that peppermint oil can relax spasms in the intestines, oesophagus and colon. Peppermint tea is one of the most commonly used herbal teas in the world.

Green tea is a popular drink made from the leaves of the Camellia sinensis plant, which is native to East Asia. It has been consumed for thousands of years and is popular for its potential health benefits, as well as its flavour and aroma. It contains several compounds, including caffeine, theanine, and catechins, that are believed to have beneficial effects. Catechins antioxidant properties help to protect cells from damage caused by free radicals. Caffeine is a stimulant that can improve alertness, mood, and cognitive performance. Theanine is an amino acid that can promote relaxation and reduce stress. The combination of caffeine and theanine in green tea is thought to enhance brain function and improve mental ability.

Other possible benefits of green tea include reducing the risk of cardiovascular disease, lowering blood pressure and cholesterol levels, improving insulin sensitivity and glucose metabolism, and reducing the risk of breast, prostate, and colorectal cancer. However, more research is needed to confirm these effects and determine the optimal dosage and duration of green tea consumption for specific health benefits.

Green tea can be consumed as a hot or cold beverage and is available in various forms, such as loose leaves, tea bags, and powdered extracts. It is generally safe for most people to consume, although high doses of green tea extract supplements may cause side effects, such as liver damage, due to the high concentration of catechins. As with other herbs and treatments, individuals taking certain medications or with certain medical conditions should consult with a healthcare provider before consuming green tea or green tea supplements.

Chapter 11
Technologies and Treatments

These days health treatments and technologies include a wide range of tools, techniques, and procedures that can be used to prevent, diagnose, monitor and treat diseases and medical conditions.

Telehealth is transforming the provision of health and well-being services and care. Remote monitoring, wireless devices, the ease with which people can communicate with doctors, nurses, physiotherapists, personal trainers, dieticians and other providers, send and receive files and images and obtain real-time video support, is revolutionising the way we access and take advantage of modern forms of health care. Appointments need not be face-to-face. Patients do not have to stay as long in hospital. Sensors and wearable devices allow constant monitoring, facilitate self-care and help ageing populations to remain independent for longer. The future is likely to be more consumer-driven and centred on lifestyle and preventive medicine. Consumers will evaluate their own bodies, use artificial intelligence diagnosis and connect with health care professionals on an ongoing or as-needed basis.

The NHS Long Term Plan states: "When ill, people will be increasingly cared for in their own home, with the option for their physiology to be effortlessly monitored by wearable devices. People will be helped to stay well, to recognise important symptoms early, and to manage their own health, guided by digital tools."

Healthcare workforces are stretched and need tools that can make patient management easier and more efficient. There are plans to increase the expansion and scaling of remote monitoring and virtual wards to free up hospital space and clinician time and accelerate the implementation of digital products.

New devices, some of which may be embedded in common household objects, will be developed. For example, how far off is a biosensing chip in a toothbrush that tracks blood sugar and bacteria levels; smart bandages that detect bacteria or a virus in a wound; smart underwear that monitors an integrated view of many vital signs; skin surface mapping that tracks changes in moles to warn of malignancies; sensing neurostimulators, assistive technologies and powered exoskeletons, respiratory support and sleep apnoea treatment, biosensors that act as portable laboratories; intelligent cochlear implants; and alternative input devices that facilitate hands-free control.

Sophisticated cars and trucks already have more than a hundred Electronic Control Units and run about 100 million lines of code. It is expected that software will become 30% of overall vehicle content. Sensors will detect drivers' and passengers' health state, emotion, attention and action. Body temperature, respiration and heart rate can be measured easily and continuously. Steering wheels may have ECG monitors. Connectivity provides options for in-car telemedicine. The vast majority of car accidents are due to human error so assessments will be made at the start of a journey and repeated periodically to track changes. Systems of infrared and 3D cameras track driver's eye movements, facial expressions, and skeletal positioning and interpret body language. The vehicle might blast the air conditioning to help a driver stay alert and propose less traffic-choked or boring routes if it perceives irritability and boredom. Driving style analysers warn of erratic behaviour. Integral breathalysers act as immobilizers. Emotion and activity software will determine if there are impairments due to fatigue, sleepiness, drugs or distractions and initiate preventative measures to avoid potential accidents. Detectors may opt for autonomous mode, slow or stop the vehicle and call for emergency help.

Let us look at some specific health and well-being technologies and treatments.

Smartwatches. Modern smartwatches offer similar functions to smartphones, they are small wearable computers in the form of a watch. They have backlit displays that are touch responsive and can connect to other devices and access calendars, emails, messages and phone calls. Many have a digital camera, altimeter, barometer and compass and include health monitoring features such as pedometer step counter, sleep pattern analysis, heartbeat tracking, ECG recording, and offer a wide range of training programs and gym workouts. Some provide rudimentary blood pressure, VO_2 Max and SpO_2 estimates. GPS tracking units are often built in which allow them to display maps and track movement, making them ideal for measuring performance in sports such as jogging and cycling. Most can be submerged underwater.

Oximeters. Pulse oximeters are reasonably inexpensive, non-invasive devices for monitoring a person's blood oxygen saturation (SpO2) which are typically within 2% accuracy. Light is beamed through the flesh and blood in a fingertip and the device measures changes in light absorption in oxygenated or deoxygenated blood. Oximeters are often used to assess lung function and monitor the health of people with conditions that affect blood oxygen levels such as: chronic obstructive pulmonary disease, asthma, pneumonia, cancer, anaemia, and heart disease.

Blood Pressure Monitors measure the pressure of blood in the arteries. Testing your blood pressure at different times of the day, especially at home, is likely to give you a more accurate understanding of your normal range of pressures than occasional visits to a doctor's clinic because 1) the stress of having the test performed in clinic can make your blood pressure go up temporarily and give a false impression when your reading is higher than usual, this effect is known as the white coat syndrome, and 2) checking more frequently also can allow you to gain a better insight into your daily routine and see the effects of events and changes in lifestyle such as your reaction to: stress, or exercise, or certain foods and drinks, or medicines.

There are two main types of blood pressure monitors: manual and digital. Manual blood pressure monitors use an inflatable cuff that is wrapped around the upper arm and a stethoscope to listen for the sounds of blood flow in the artery. The cuff is inflated until it stops blood flow and then slowly deflated while a healthcare provider listens. The first sound they hear indicates the systolic pressure; the second sound indicates the diastolic pressure. Digital blood pressure monitors are automated and do not require a stethoscope. They use an electronic sensor to detect the pressure of blood flow in the artery and display the readings on a screen.

The most accurate digital monitors use upper arm inflatable cuffs. Some are capable of storing multiple readings and calculating an average over time.

Weighing scales and smart body composition monitors. Bathroom scales have come a long way. Modern digital weighing scales provide far more information than accurate estimates of a person's weight. These devices often have metal or conductive plates such that, when an individual stands on the scale in bare feet, mild electrical signals are sent through the body that measure transmission / resistance and, from that, assumptions are made that allow calculations of parameters such as: body fat, BMI, lean mass, muscle mass, bone mass, visceral fat, and hydration. They use Bio Impedance Analysis, technology that passes tiny electrical impulses through the body to estimate amounts of fat and lean tissue. Some include extra sensors that are held in the hands. Many modern bathroom scales are designed to be wirelessly or cellularly connected and have features like smartphone integration, cloud storage, and fitness tracking.

DNA Genetic Testing. Genetic testing may provide diagnosis of a person's vulnerabilities to inherited diseases and can be used to determine ancestry. Our DNA is passed down to us from our parents. Human DNA is about 99.5% identical from person to person. Small differences, called variants, make each person unique. Genotyping looks at specific DNA locations (known to be associated with important health conditions, ancestry and traits) and identifies variants. The results of a genetic test can help to confirm or rule out a suspected genetic condition or estimate a person's chance of developing or passing on a genetic disorder. Genetic testing can identify changes in chromosomes, genes, or proteins and is often used to find changes that are associated with inherited disorders.

Blood Tests. Cholesterol and blood glucose test kits are used to measure, or give an indication of, the amount of cholesterol or glucose (sugar) in a person's blood. There are a wide variety of home cholesterol and blood glucose test kits (sampling kits) available for sale online and in pharmacies. They vary in quality and reliability and may not be as accurate as a lab-based test but they can be useful in assessing and monitoring levels.

The kits often include lancets, test strips and meters with digital displays. Glucose meters are small electronic devices that measure the amount of glucose in a small drop of blood. The lancet is a small, sharp needle that is used to prick the skin and draw blood, and the test strips are inserted into the glucose meter to measure the amount of glucose in the blood sample. Home cholesterol testing kits will only give a total cholesterol estimate. A random blood test is a test that is taken without the need to fast beforehand.

Alternatively you can choose to send a blood sample off to firms that offers to do the testing for you, for a variety of different conditions (from bone and muscle health through to thyroid, liver and kidney function tests and heart disease risks). Samples that are sent to a laboratory are likely to be more accurate and trustworthy and give a fuller breakdown. Results are usually available within a week or so.

An ApoB test seems to be a useful way to assess our risk for heart disease. It measures the amount of apolipoprotein B, which is the main protein found in low-density lipoproteins (LDL). LDL cholesterol is more frequently measured than ApoB levels because it's included as part of a standard cholesterol test. Emerging research indicates that ApoB is an indicator of heart health, heart disease risk and plaque build-up in our blood vessels.

Continuous Glucose Monitors let us keep an eye on our sugar levels all day without having to prick our fingers. Until recently the only way to know your glucose levels was to puncture you skin a few times a day and take a measure in a drop of blood. Whilst finger pricking assesses the current glucose level at the time, it does not tell us where glucose levels are heading or how quickly, and does not provide a full picture of daily ups and downs and what affects us. People get sore fingers and grow frustrated at being unable to predict hypoglycaemia and hyperglycaemia, or keep their glucose in range. Continuous glucose monitoring (CGM) systems, measure glucose levels every 5 minutes, letting people see how their glucose levels are changing over time. A small sensor, worn 24 hours a day, monitors levels and transmits data to a phone and possibly to a parent, carer or healthcare provider. An alarm can be set to sound if levels go too low or too high. Charts and graphs provide valuable and informative ways to see and understand how food, activity, stress and other variables affect our sugar levels. This technology is not only useful to people with diabetes, CGMs are being used more and more as revealing health and wellbeing tracking devices.

Urine tests are easy to perform, non-invasive, inexpensive and can signal certain common diseases. Urinalysis can be used to detect problems that need treatment before we feel symptoms or they get worse, including infections, kidney disease, diabetes, and liver disease. Kits can be bought on-line or from pharmacies. A plastic dipstick, with strips of chemicals on it, is dipped into a sample of urine. The strips change colour if a substance is present at a level that is above normal such as: 1) acidity – high pH may be a sign of kidney stones, urinary infections, kidney problems, or other disorders. 2) protein - which should only be in our blood, not our urine. When our kidneys are injured, protein may leak into our urine so having protein in our urine can suggest that our kidney's filtering units are damaged. 3) Glucose – which is often a sign of diabetes. 4) White blood cells (pus cells) are signs of infection. 5) Bilirubin is a waste product from the breakdown of old red blood cells which is normally removed from the blood by the liver, so its presence in the urine may be a sign of liver disease. 6) Blood can be a sign of an infection, a kidney problem, the result of certain medicines, or even heavy exercise. Finding blood in the urine requires further testing but does not mean we have a serious medical problem.

Faecal matter transplant (FMT) is a medical procedure in which faecal matter from a healthy donor is transplanted into the colon of a patient who is suffering from certain conditions. The purpose of the transplant is to introduce healthy gut bacteria from the donor into the recipient's gut, in order to restore the natural balance of gut microbiota. FMT is most commonly used to treat recurrent Clostridium Difficile Infection (CDI). It has also been explored as a potential treatment for other conditions such as inflammatory bowel disease, irritable bowel syndrome, and even neurological disorders like Parkinson's disease.

Luxury smart toilets offer an astonishing list of features and functions including: LED lights; lids that have motion sensors so they lift automatically when they are approached; heated seats for optimum comfort, some models even feature a massage setting; a built-in bidet so that users can benefit from more hygienic cleaning after toilet use; remote-controlled shower jet, some come equipped with a "lady shower" function;

automated cleaning technology, the toilet cleans itself automatically after every use; a 5 speed warm air dryer that operates once the shower jet has finished, the temperature and pressures can be adjusted to suit personal preference and be saved for next time; auto flush when the user stands up; a deodoriser to absorb any smells using a bamboo charcoal filter; a stop function which can be used at any time to stop the washing and air-drying functions; a night light in case you struggle to find the toilet in the dark and the main light is too bright; energy saving, the toilet can be placed on standby to reduce your carbon footprint; and music, some toilets include the option to play music to help the user relax or to act as a masking sound to spare blushes.

Using sensors and artificial intelligence to analyse waste, the loo could become a common household health monitoring tool. Our stool and urine samples can be used to track our outputs, our risk of disease, our diet, our microbiome, our calorie intake, our exercise level; how much alcohol we drink and whether we take drugs. It may analyse samples continually to detect signs of pregnancy, diabetes and cancer. Having technology that tracks what is normal for an individual (a healthy baseline) will help to provide an early warning if a check-up is needed, so these toilets may provide peace of mind for many people. To differentiate between users, scanners may be used that can recognise the physical characteristics of whoever is sitting on the toilet, including, apparently, our "analprint", which, like our fingerprints, is unique.

This innovative technology is fraught with ethical concerns. For example, to what extent and in what circumstances might parents, employers, insurance companies and the police gain access to this data?

Whole-body vibration seems to offer benefits to some people, especially those who find it difficult to exercise. Individuals stand or sit on a vibrating platform which transmits energy to the body and makes muscles contract and relax multiple times per minute. Advocates suggest that about 15 minutes a day of whole-body vibration, three times a week, may aid weight loss, burn fat, improve flexibility, enhance blood flow, reduce muscle soreness after exercise, build strength and decrease the stress hormone cortisol, but there is little conclusive evidence to back all this up. Some research indicates that whole-body vibration may help to improve muscle strength and that, when performed correctly it can reduce back pain and improve balance in older adults. Although generally safe, whole-body vibration may be harmful, so people with ill health should consult with their doctor before using it, especially if they are pregnant or have health problems.

Ultrasound. Ultrasonic transducer probes for medical and thera-peutic use come in a variety of different shapes and sizes. Ultrasound has several advantages when compared to other medical imaging tech-nologies. It provides real-time, dynamic images, it is substantially less expensive and it does not use harmful ionizing radiation. Wearable ultra-sound implementations are gaining popularity. These miniature devices continuously monitor vitals and alert at the emergence of early signs of abnormality. There are also ultrasound treatment devices that are said to accelerate healing and reduce the need for pain medication and surgery. The ultrasound radiates directly into tissue approximately 5 cm deep and can achieve a therapeutic dosing area that is about the size of an orange. Many of these products carry safety warnings.

Massage Therapy is one of the earliest known therapies, it was used by several ancient cultures, including the Greeks, Egyptians, Chinese, and Indians. It can be a powerful tool to enhance your overall health and well-being. It can relax you, reduce your stress and tension, lower your heart rate and blood pressure, improve your circulation, reduce pain and muscle soreness, eliminate certain toxins, improve your flexibility and sleep, and enhance your immunity. You should avoid getting a massage if you: have cancer or fractures or inflammation or a fever, contagious disease, infection or internal bleeding or blood clots, are pregnant, have problems with your liver or kidneys, or have uncontrolled hypertension.

Sauna use is thought to be good for your healthy life expectancy. Researchers report reduced risk of sudden cardiac death, fatal coronary heart disease, fatal cardiovascular disease, and all-cause mortality in sauna users. The saunas' dry heat (which can get as high as 85° C) has quite profound effects on our body. Our skin temperature rises quickly to about 40°C and we may sweat 500ml or more. Our pulse rate is likely to jump, allowing our heart to increase the amount of blood it pumps each minute, most of which is directed to the skin. Saunas appear to be safe for most people, however, those with uncontrolled high blood pressure and heart disease should check with their doctors before entering one.

Sensible precautions include: stay in no more than 20 minutes, drink lots of water after each sauna; avoid alcohol and medications that may impair sweating and produce overheating before and after your sauna, and do not take a sauna when you are ill.

Ice Baths and Cold Water Therapy. Ice baths are used by some athletes after a period of intense exercise to help with recovery. A brief ice bath seems to soothe muscles, reduce inflammation, improve breathing, and give you a boost. Cold water therapy is thought to be beneficial because it constricts blood vessels, reduces swelling and tissue breakdown and flushes out waste products. Afterwards, as the tissues warm and the increased blood flow speeds circulation, the healing process may be jump started. Ice baths are said to be better than ice packs because they submerge most of the body rather than a small patch. However, the method is controversial, there is a risk of cardiac shock and hypothermia and evidence supporting cold water immersion remains inconclusive.

Red light therapy may help skin, muscle tissue, and other parts of the body repair themselves and heal. It gives low levels of red light (that you can see) or near-infrared light, (energy that your eyes can not see, but your body feels as heat). Red light is thought to work by producing a biochemical effect that strengthens the mitochondria which are the powerhouse of cells. Many laboratory and clinical studies have been conducted to determine if red light therapy has medical benefits. Some have had promising results, but this treatment is still a source of controversy and there is not enough convincing evidence to show that these devices are better than other ways of treating wounds, ulcers, and pain.

Some light therapy boxes mimic outdoor light because it is thought that this type of light may cause chemical changes in the brain that lift your mood and ease other symptoms of Seasonal Affective Disorder (SAD), such as being tired most of the time and sleeping too much.

Acupuncture is part of traditional Chinese medicine. It uses very fine needles which are gently inserted through the skin at specific places and left in position for a short while. Traditional acupuncture is based on the principle that a life force called Qi (pronounced 'chee') runs along energy channels in the body called meridians. It is thought that one's health is negatively affected when the flow of Qi is interrupted and that inserting needles can restore the flow and return the body to health. Practitioners of Western medical acupuncture suggest that the beneficial effects come as a result of directly stimulating nerves and muscles which prompt the release of natural substances into the body such as endorphins that relieve stress and pain. Acupuncture is safe for most people, unless you have an allergy to certain metals or a blood clotting disorder or are taking blood thinning medication.

Shiatsu is a non-invasive physical therapy originating from Japan. It uses a combination of kneading, pressing, tapping and stretching techniques which can reduce tension and re-energise the body. The Japanese Ministry of Health defines shiatsu as "a form of manipulation by thumbs, fingers and palms without the use of instruments, mechanical or otherwise, to apply pressure to the human skin to correct internal malfunctions, promote and maintain health, and treat specific diseases". Like Acupuncture, Shiatsu is said to work with the body's energy flow, known as Ki or Qi, and treat the functioning of nervous, circulatory and respiratory systems. It supports the body's innate self-healing abilities and promotes a sense of relaxation and well-being. Shiatsu harmonizes and supports our overall energy and addresses imbalances which could manifest on a physical and / or emotional level. Research indicates that Shiatsu is safe and may reduce a wide range of symptoms, improve quality of life decrease dependency on medication.

The Hand Grip Strength Test. A person's overall strength can be quantified to a surprisingly accurate extent by measuring the amount of static force that their left or right hand can squeeze around a handheld dynamometer. Grip strength is a measure of muscular strength or the maximum force/tension generated by one's forearm muscles. It is a standard, useful and reliable measurement which is predictive of certain health conditions and can be used as a screening tool for the measurement of overall strength.

Spirometers measure the amount of air you can breathe out in one second and the total volume of air you can exhale in one forced breath. Spirometry is a simple test used to help diagnose and monitor certain lung conditions. It measures the volume of air inspired and expired by the lungs. A spirometer measures ventilation, the movement of air into and out of the lungs. The spirogram will identify two different types of abnormal ventilation patterns, obstructive and restrictive.

The Quantitative Digitography (QDG) team has developed a unique approach to managing Parkinson's Disease by using a repetitive alternating finger-tapping (RAFT) task on the redesigned KeyDuo device and a proprietary algorithm (PRECISE), which has been demonstrated to accurately and robustly measure and monitor the core motor signs of Parkinson's Disease. Using a remote device-based approach, the team has developed a monitoring and diagnostic system to inform patients and physicians about the control and management of the patient's chronic condition, with the intention of expanding access to neurological care. Remote measurements and monitoring provide reliable data for the health care provider that will improve treatment and reduce or prevent complications of therapy. The QDG team plans to provide access to the patient's data from their chart in the Electronic Health Record, enabling health care providers to easily access this data and make complex treatment decisions. The team has published multiple studies and performed clinical trials demonstrating QDG's efficacy and has patented, engineered, and designed a prototype device and proprietary algorithm.

Artificial intelligence (AI) and digital technologies are being employed to improve healthcare delivery and patient outcomes. AI health applications include diagnosis and treatment recommendations, patient monitoring and management, drug development, and personalized medicine. AI health tools can help healthcare professionals to analyse large amounts of data, identify patterns and anomalies, and make faster and more accurate diagnoses. They can also help patients to manage chronic conditions, monitor their own health, and receive personalized treatment recommendations.

It is likely that AI will be used more and more to provide information on health-related topics, such as symptoms, treatments, and preventive measures to help people make informed decisions about their health and well-being. AI has the potential to change peoples' health and well-being in numerous ways by providing accessible, personalized, and accurate health information, promoting healthy habits, and advancing medical research. For example:

- Mental health support and advice to people who may be experiencing anxiety, depression, or other mental health conditions.

- Assistance in diagnosing and managing diseases by analysing symptoms and providing treatment recommendations.

- Encouraging healthy habits by offering guidance and motivation to help people adopt healthy habits, such as exercising regularly, eating a balanced diet, and getting enough sleep.

- Analysing large amounts of medical data to help researchers identify patterns and make new discoveries in the field of medicine, which could lead to the development of new treatments and therapies.

However, the use of AI in healthcare also raises ethical and regulatory concerns around data privacy, bias, and accountability. As with any new technology, it is important to evaluate the benefits and risks of AI health applications carefully and ensure that they are developed and used responsibly.

Chapter 12

Conclusions

Given the rising levels of chronic diseases, worryingly low Healthy Life Expectancies (HLEs), pandemic after effects and pressures on health services, there are many reasons to suggest that everyone needs to become more aware of, and take more responsibility for looking after, their health and well-being. We must learn to keep an eye on, test and monitor important factors and indicators. The **More From Life** approach provides a way to do this.

Lifestyle medicine attempts to prevent and treat the causes of chronic diseases. We have already noted that if everyone just did four reasonably simple things: (not smoking, exercising a half hour a day, eating a diet that is based on whole plant foods, and not becoming obese), we could prevent most cases of diabetes and heart attacks, half of strokes, and a third of cancers. Even modest changes may be more effective in reducing cardiovascular disease, high blood pressure, heart failure, stroke, cancer, diabetes, and all-cause mortality than almost any other medical intervention. The key difference between conventional medicine and lifestyle medicine is, instead of just treating risk factors, we treat the underlying causes of disease. For example, high blood pressure is often a symptom of diseased and dysfunctional arteries. Taking drugs for half a lifetime, to lower high blood pressure artificially, does not treat the underlying cause, instead we should try to encourage changes in habits of diet and exercise.

Systemic Approach

So, there is strong evidence that lifestyle factors are important consid-erations in healthcare, but how easy is it to assess someone's overall health and well-being status? Plus, how do we notice and track signif-icant changes and developments? It seems clear there is a need for an inexpensive, systemic health and wellbeing evaluation and monitoring approach, especially these days as so many danger or warning signs are being missed. A useful health promotion and monitoring approach would be likely to enhance peoples' wellbeing as well as alerting them to signs of ill-health.

Many people are keen to monitor and track aspects of their fitness and health. Most of the tools that help them to do this only provide limited amounts of data such as their: weight, steps per day, calorie intake, approximate heart rate and hours of sleep. Few if any cover a broad range that includes nutrition / diet, physical strength and fitness, medical health and mental well-being.

An approach that is systemic offers a richer picture. One that allows people to gauge, quantify and measure many different indicators of their health and wellbeing can be beneficial as it can: provide quantifiable and graphical feedback that can be tracked week by week or month by month; highlight aspects that may be changing, or concerning or need attention; assist with the prevention and reversal of illness; and give incentive and direction that encourages healthier living.

More From Life aims to promote and encourage personalised strategies for monitoring and improving aspects of health. It invites people to take a set of assessments under the broad headings of: Body, Mind, Nutrition and Fitness / Exercise. The **One Week Challenge** provides a straightfor-ward, directed approach to measuring before and after status, in a short timescale that should show gratifying and encouraging improvements and lead to longer term challenges and good habits.

More From Life assessments can be taken as often as convenient. Having done the tests and questions in the 5 sections that make up the 500 points, people can go back and try certain parts (the parts they want to concentrate on, retest or improve) again, updating their overall score each time.

Participants should remember that if they feel any unusual discomfort in their chest, arm, jaw, shoulders or between their shoulder blades while exercising they should consult a doctor or health professional. If any of the functional movement tests or other exercise assessments cause pain (rather than muscle burn) they should discuss this with a health professional or physiotherapist.

While the **More From Life One Week Challenge** assesses many aspects of a person's health and well-being, it does not attempt to cover or take into account every factor or consideration that may affect a person's health and well-being such as:

Check-ups for:

- Teeth and gums.
- Eyes / eyesight.
- Ears / Hearing.
- Skin / moles, irritating rashes and melanoma.
- Unusual signs of bleeding.
- Difficulty beathing.
- Pain, numbness or unusual tingling in limbs.
- Breasts, testicles, swellings, lumps and bumps.
- Coughs that last 3 weeks or more.
- Deep depression and anxiety.
- Sudden unexplained changes.

Other Important Issues

To a great extent, people's underlying health depends on environmental factors many of which are largely out of their control, such as: where they grow up, live and work, their housing, what education they get, what their income is, whether they have good social support networks and their culture and beliefs.

- Genetics plays a part in determining lifespan, healthiness and the likelihood of developing certain illnesses.

- People employed in good working conditions are healthier, particularly those who have more control over their work.
- Higher incomes and social status are linked to better health.
- Low education levels are linked with poor health, more stress and lower self-confidence.
- Customs and traditions, plus support from families, friends and communities all affect health.
- Access to, and use of, health services that help to prevent and treat disease.

Deprivation and poverty: studies indicate that people in the most deprived areas have shorter lives and spend around a third of their lives in poor health, (twice the proportion spent by those in the least deprived areas). Women born in the least deprived areas not only live 10 years longer on average, but also tend to benefit from 21.5 more years in good health. Poverty is linked with negative conditions such as substandard housing, homelessness, poor and inadequate nutrition, food insecurity, inadequate child care, lack of access to health care, unsafe neighborhoods, and under-resourced schools. Research has shown that lower socio-economic status and neighbourhood deprivation are associated with premature mortality, increased incidence of psychosis, mental health service use, coronary heart disease, and behavioural problems in children and adolescents. Poverty has negative impacts on children's health, social, emotional and cognitive development, behaviour and educational outcomes. Children born into poverty are more likely to experience a wide range of health problems, disease and mental health problems.

Education: the contribution of education to long-term health has been described as offering both protection and potential. It can prompt healthier futures, mitigate social problems, and provide access to employment opportunities and life opportunities that could protect many individuals from later-life disadvantage. Education is known to be one of the most important, modifiable determinants of health. Studies show that the more educated and skilled we are, the more likely we will have better health even when compared with people with similar backgrounds. A good education tends to reduce lifetime stress levels, and helps us to access well-paid and satisfying employment, live in safer and healthier environments, develop an attitude and aptitude for life-long learning and problem solving, feel more empowered and valued, create healthy habits and build strong foundations for supportive social connections.

Addiction is defined as not having control over doing, taking or using something to the point where it starts to dominate our lives and may become harmful. Being addicted means that not having something causes withdrawal symptoms. Addiction is commonly associated with drugs, gambling, alcohol and smoking. Unemployment and poverty can trigger addiction, along with stress, emotional and professional pressure. Addiction can have dramatic physical and psychological effects and, in some cases, can be a devastating disease, with a relatively high death rate and serious social consequences. People with addictions may behave destructively, they may crave and try to obtain more drugs, alcohol, or other substances no matter what the cost, even at the risk of hurting their family, friends, or health, or losing jobs. There is a widespread misunderstanding that addiction is a choice, that all any addict has to do is stop, but addiction often causes changes in the brain and it may take a great deal of effort and help to return someone who has an addiction to a happier and healthier state.

Environmental factors. Poor air quality is thought to be the largest environmental risk to public health in the UK. Long-term exposure to air pollution can cause chronic conditions such as cardiovascular and respiratory diseases, leading to reduced life expectancy. When air pollutants enter the body, they can have negative effects on various organs, including the eyes, nose and throat, the lungs and the heart. Evidence suggests that air pollution can also affect the brain and may be linked to dementia and cognitive decline. Even quite short-term exposure to elevated levels of air pollution can cause a range of health impacts, including exacerbation of asthma, increases in respiratory and cardiovascular hospital admissions and mortality.

Air pollution is a complex mix that usually includes particulate matter and nitrogen dioxide (NO_2). The main sources of man-made particulate matter in urban areas are fuel combustion and tyre and brake wear. Natural sources include dust and fires. The size of particles and the duration of exposure are key determinants of adverse health effects. Larger particles may be deposited in the nose or throat, smaller particles can pose greater risk because they are drawn deeper into the lungs.

Noise pollution affects millions of people. The most common health problem it may cause is hearing loss but exposure to loud noise can also cause high blood pressure, heart disease, sleep disturbances, and stress. These health problems can affect all age groups, especially children.

Plastic pollution threatens the environment, our health and that of future generations. Humans are exposed to an astonishing variety of toxic chemicals and microplastics through inhalation, ingestion, and direct skin contact. It has been estimated that we ingest about 5 grams of plastic every week. Scientific research to-date indicates that the toxic chemical additives and pollutants found in plastics threaten human, marine and land animal and plant health on a global scale. Some of the effects on us are known to include endocrine disruption, (which can lead to reproductive, growth, and cognitive impairment) and certain cancers.

Even small amounts of exposure to mercury can cause quite serious health problems, it may have toxic effects on our nervous, digestive and immune systems, and on our lungs, kidneys, skin and eyes. Mercury is considered by the WHO to be one of the top 10 chemicals of major public health concern (along with Arsenic, Asbestos, Benzene, Cadmium, Dioxin, Lead and hazardous Pesticides). People are more likely to consume methylmercury when they eat fish such as tuna and swordfish.

Dioxins are highly toxic and can cause reproductive and developmental problems, damage the immune system, interfere with hormones and cause cancer. They are found throughout the world in the environment and they accumulate in the food chain, mainly in the fatty tissue of animals, so more than 90% of human exposure is through food, mainly meat and dairy products, fish and shellfish. The higher an animal is in the food chain, the higher the concentration of dioxins. Once dioxins enter the body, they can last a long time.

Laughter. The old saying that "laughter is the best medicine" rings true. Having fun and a laugh with friends and family is known to be good for us in many ways. Laughter triggers the release of endorphins, the body's natural feel-good chemicals that reduce stress, promote an overall sense of well-being and can relieve pain. Laughter strengthens the immune system and improves our resistance to disease. It is good for our heart. When we laugh our blood vessels dilate allowing the blood to flow more easily and lower our blood pressure. Laughter can also help us when it comes to our personal relationships, not only with people we already know and feel comfortable with, but with strangers and those we hardly know, as well. It draws people together in ways that trigger healthy physical and emotional changes in the body. It helps to alleviate feelings of fear and rage. A sense of humour can dissipate negative emotions such as anger and aggression and laughter can calm tense and difficult situations and clear the air.

Recommended Resources

A number of authoritative and highly credible authors deserve mention and provide deeper explanation and scientific evidence of many of the suggestions and issues discussed in this book. They include:

- Dean Ornish – "*Undo It!: How Simple Lifestyle Changes Can Reverse Most Chronic Diseases*", and "*The Spectrum*".

- Michael Greger – "*How Not To Die*", and "*How not to Diet*".

- Caldwell Esselstyn – "*Prevent And Reverse Heart Disease: The Revolutionary, Scientifically Proven, Nutrition-Based Cure*".

- Neal Barnard – "*Reversing Diabetes: The Scientifically Proven System for Reversing Diabetes Without Drugs*", and "*The Vegan Starter Kit*", and "*21 Day Weight Loss Kickstart*", and "*Your Body In Balance: The New Science of Food, Hormones and Health*".

- Shireen Kassam - "*Eating Plant-Based: Scientific Answers to Your Nutrition Questions*" and "*Plant-Based Nutrition in Clinical Practice*".

- Tim Spector – "*Spoon Fed*" and "*Food For Life, The New Science Of Eating Well*".

- Brooke Goldner – "*Goodbye Lupus: How a Medical Doctor Healed Herself Naturally With Supermarket Foods*" and "*Goodbye Autoimmune Disease: How to Prevent and Reverse*

Chronic Illness and Inflammatory Symptoms Using Supermarket Foods".

- Peter Attia and Bill Gifford – *"Outlive: The Science and Art of Longevity".*
- Ancel Keys and Margaret Keys – *"The Benevolent Bean"* and *"How to Eat Well and Stay Well the Mediterranean Way".*

All of the above authors are medical doctors and most have conducted careful well-documented, research for many years.

Other Authors worthy of mention:

- T Colin Campbell – *"The China Study: The Most Comprehensive Study of Nutrition Ever Conducted and the Startling Implications for Diet, Weight Loss, and Long-Term Health".*
- John Robbins – *"Healthy at 100: The Scientifically Proven Secrets of the World's Healthiest and Longest-Lived Peoples".*
- Herman Pontzer – *"Burn: New Research Blows the Lid Off How We Really Burn Calories, Stay Healthy, and Lose Weight".*
- Nathan Pritikin – *"The Pritikin Program for Diet and Exercise"* and *"The Pritikin Promise: 28 Days to a Longer, Healthier Life".*
- Pamela A. Popper – *"Food over Medicine: The Conversation That Could Save Your Life"*, and *"Food Choices: Eat Better, Live Better and Help Save the Planet".*
- Elaine R Ingham – *The Soil Food Web School.*
- Richard A. Oppenlander – *"Comfortably Unaware: Global Depletion and Food Responsibility, What You Choose To Eat is Killing Our Planet".*
- Rich Roll – *"Finding Ultra, Rejecting Middle Age, Becoming One of the World's Fittest Men, and Discovering Myself".*
- Brendan Brazier – *"Thrive: The Plant-Based Whole Foods Way to Staying Healthy for Life".*
- Dan Buettner – *"The Blue Zones Solution: Eating and Living Like the World's Healthiest People".*
- Juliet Starrett and Kelly Starrett - *"Built to Move"*

There is a song with the same name as this book, *"More Life"*, written by Mike Reid and Rory Bourke and sung by Randy Travis and Don Henley (recorded in 2011).

Several films and documentaries have highlighted issues mentioned in this book, including: *Forks Over Knives; The Game Changers; What the Health; Fat, Sick and Nearly Dead; Living Soil; Eating Our Way to Extinction; Cowspiracy; Seaspiracy; Dominion; From the Ground Up; Eating You Alive; Kiss the Ground.*

YouTubers: *NutritionFacts, Plant Based Health Professionals, Michael Kalper, Gemma Newman, Plant Chompers, Physicians Committee for Responsible Medicine, The Happy Pear, Dr. John Campbell, Nutrition Made Simple.*

Final Words

Life is a complex and multifaceted experience, full of ups and downs, surprises and routines, joys and sorrows, triumphs and fails. It is a journey that is unique to each individual shaped by their attitudes, well-being, abilities, training, interactions, beliefs, values, and perspectives. We learn and grow, develop new skills and perspectives, discover new passions, interests, and talents, and face new challenges. Strong and healthy relationships with family, friends, romantic partners, and colleagues are built on trust, communication, respect, and understanding. They play a critical role in shaping who we are and provide us with the support, love, and encouragement we need to navigate our lives. We all encounter struggles and setbacks, health issues, financial difficulties and personal crises that demand effort, strength and resilience. We draw on our inner resources and support networks in our efforts to overcome these challenges and emerge stronger, happier and more confident than before, achieving **More From Life**.

We have looked at ways to sustain, amplify and promote both life-span and health-span in this book. To increase our life-span we need to take steps to prevent and delay the onset of common killers such as diabetes, cardiovascular disease and cancer as long as possible. To improve and extend our health-span we need to look after our brain (cognitive decline and dementia), our emotional health (having purpose, social relationships and avoiding depression) and our physical health (maintaining mobility, strength, bone and muscle density, aerobic ability, flexibility, sexual function and freedom from pain).

To appreciate and maintain our health and well-being we should monitor a wide variety of indicators. By measuring different aspects regularly we can gain insight into potential problems and disease risks and make informed decisions about how to improve our current status.

Adhering to just five healthy lifestyle factors has a strong impact on the prevention of chronic diseases and increases our chances of living longer:

1. walking and getting 30 minutes of exercise a day,
2. not smoking,
3. not being overweight,
4. maintaining happy relationships (your social fitness) and
5. eating a healthy diet (defined as more fruit, veg and whole grains and far less meat).

Studies show that adopting these lifestyle changes can increase life expectancy by 12 to 14 years. If you tick all five you can reduce your risk of getting diabetes by 90%, your risk of a heart attack by 80%, your risk of a stoke by 50% and your risk of many cancers by about 35% (71% for colon cancer).

You do not need to adopt every recommendation in this book, it does not have to be all or nothing. If you do not have heart disease you can afford to stray from the path, … occasionally! The more you move in a healthful direction the more likely you are to look and feel better, be happier, smell and taste better, be stronger, move better, lose unwanted body fat and gain health.

Food is medicine, you need to eat a well-balanced vegetarian or flexitarian diet to stay well and help your body heal itself. What we consume is the number one cause of disability and premature death. Avoid processed food. Eat colourful, whole, organic, plant-based produce. Stay active most of the day, go for walks and do some regular strength training. Bear in mind the environmental and animal welfare impacts of your food choices. Keep in touch with your friends and family and be generous every day. Find time to relax and rest. If you do not get much exercise or over indulge yourself one day, make up for it the next. Track the **More From Life** indicators and measurements to keep an eye on your health and wellbeing.

You can also help other people to become happier and healthier.

Ancient Chinese proverb:
"We have two lives, the second begins when
we realise we only have one."
— Confucius

Get More From Life.

About the Author

The son of a cardiologist and an ophthalmologist Malcolm Bronte-Stewart grew up in a medical family and follows developments in lifestyle medicine. Graduating from Aberdeen University, he worked on a horse ranch in Canada, as a canoe expedition leader in Wales, a ski instructor in France and outdoor sports organiser in the highlands of Scotland before becoming the Director of Endeavour Training, an outward-bound school. He went on to work as a geologist then retrained as a systems analyst consultant before becoming a university lecturer for over 30 years, publishing research on Systems Thinking, Project Management, Rich Pictures, Information Systems Consultancy and the Life Number experiment. He and his wife manage a farm and equitation centre.

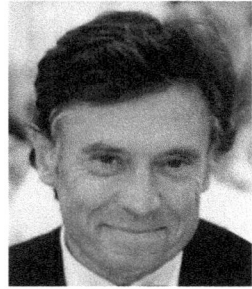

You can contact Malcolm at:

Instagram: morefromlifehealth

Facebook: More From Life

www.ingramcontent.com/pod-product-compliance
Lightning Source LLC
Chambersburg PA
CBHW051258020426
42333CB00026B/3254